Critical Care Intravenous Infusion Drug Handbook

Second Edition

Gary J. Algozzine, PharmD, BCNSP
Director of Pharmacy
Blake Medical Center
Bradenton, Florida
Assistant Clinical Professor, College of Pharmacy
University of Florida
Gainesville, Florida

Robert Algozzine, PhD
Professor, College of Education
Department of Educational Leadership
The University of North Carolina at Charlotte
Charlotte, North Carolina

Deborah J. Lilly, RN, MSN, CCRN
Clinical Nurse Specialist
Critical Care Training and Development
Blake Medical Center
Bradenton, Florida

ELSEVIER
MOSBY

ELSEVIER
MOSBY

11830 Westline Industrial Drive
St. Louis, Missouri 63146

CRITICAL CARE INTRAVENOUS INFUSION DRUG HANDBOOK, SECOND EDITION   0-323-03121-8

Notice

Critical care is an ever-changing field. Standard safety precautions must be followed, but as new research and clinical experience broaden our knowledge, changes in treatment and drug therapy may become necessary or appropriate. Readers are advised to check the most current product information provided by the manufacturer of each drug to be administered to verify the recommended dose, the method and duration of administration, and contraindications. It is the responsibility of the licensed prescriber, relying on experience and knowledge of the patient, to determine dosages and the best treatment for each individual patient. Neither the publisher nor the author assumes any liability for any injury and/or damage to persons or property arising from this publication.

Previous edition copyrighted 2002.

International Standard Book Number: 0-323-03121-8

Executive Publisher: Barbara Nelson Cullen
Developmental Editor: Julie Vitale
Publishing Services Manager: Deborah L. Vogel
Senior Project Manager: Ann E. Rogers
Cover and Interior Designer: Amy Buxton

Printed in the United States of America
Last digit is the print number: 9 8 7 6 5 4 3 2 1

This work is dedicated to the memory of Nicholas and Jennie Algozzine. Their love, support, and guidance enriched everyone they touched, and without them this book would not be possible. Nothing is a stronger influence on the success of children than the continuing gift of wonderful parents.

Reviewers

Patricia Harris, RN, BSN, CCRN
Children's Hospital of Pittsburgh
Pittsburgh, Pennsylvania

Maureen A. Seckel, RN, APN, MSN, CCRN, CS
Christian Care Health Services
Newark, Delaware

Susan C. Vaughan, RN, BSN
Carolinas Medical Center
Charlotte, North Carolina

Preface

Each day thousands of people are administered critical care drugs to correct or stabilize complicated medical conditions associated with acute and chronic illness. These drugs are not easy to administer and often require sophisticated dosing regimens. Healthcare professionals require the use of drug references to assist them and ensure the safe, effective, and correct administration of these complex drugs.

Decisions associated with critical care treatment have a profound effect on the well-being of patients and the respect and reputation of caregivers. The *Critical Care Intravenous Infusion Drug Handbook*, second edition, is a resource for this critical medical practice. It is a practical handbook for hospital critical care nurses, pharmacists, and physicians, containing information on how to dose and administer 44 commonly used complex critical care drugs. Each drug in this handbook is listed with information about its most common uses, how to prepare the drug infusion for patient administration, the most common dosages (including a dosing chart, when appropriate), the most common warnings and adverse reactions, compatibility with other drug infusions, and general nursing considerations. Because most of these drugs are dosed by patient weight, when appropriate, each dosing chart contains the dose in micrograms per kilogram per minute and the corresponding infusion rate to deliver this dose. When appropriate, calculation factors are listed for each patient weight. These calculation factors are used by nurses to quickly change a patient's infusion dose and titrate the drug to the desired physiologic response, such as blood pressure. This information is used on a daily basis with many patients and until now was not available in this easy-to-use format.

The primary audience for the *Critical Care Intravenous Infusion Drug Handbook* is critical care nurses, such as those who work in hospital intensive care units, coronary care units, operating rooms, postanesthesia area units, open heart surgery units, and emergency departments. This book is also of use to general medicine or general surgical nurses in settings where these drugs are commonly administered, as well as hospital pharmacists and physicians, who are responsible for mixing and ordering these drugs, respectively. Critical care physicians, cardiologists, anesthesiologists, and emergency room physicians will find the information provided in this handbook of great value when prescribing these drugs. In addition, a copy of the *Critical Care Intravenous Infusion Drug Handbook* should be on every Code Blue Crash Cart for use during cardiac arrest.

The most unique features of this book are the ease of use and the dosing charts for what are complicated drugs to administer. Its format allows the healthcare professional to quickly determine how to mix and prepare drugs that are usually needed by the patient on an immediate, urgent basis, and the dosing charts allow the nursing staff to determine the appropriate dose in a matter of seconds. Having calculation factors for drugs is very practical. These charts alone greatly simplify an otherwise complicated process and substantially reduce the chance for dosage errors.

The information in this handbook provides guidelines for administration of commonly prescribed intravenous (IV) infusion medications. The intent is to provide a guide to support quality patient care with regard to the clinical use of specific drugs in hospital settings. Each dosing chart lists the drug concentration that should match the concentration of the actual drug, bottle, or infusion being administered to the patient. The guidelines provided are for general adult patients and are not intended for pediatric or pregnant patients. We have attempted to include only common drugs that are administered by intravenous infusion and often require complex dosing and infusion regimens. The information is not intended to replace the reasoned nursing or clinical judgment of qualified professional personnel on a case-by-case basis. Specific hospital-based protocols and policies should be followed and may differ from recommendations in this text. In almost all cases, most of these drugs should be administered using some type of controlled infusion pump, many of which have preprogrammed multiple safeguards, such as "guard rails" or "guardian" features to assist staff and safeguard patients. Questions and concerns regarding provision of care related to these medications should be referred to supervisory staff members, pharmacy professionals, and/or the appropriate physician for review, guidance, and direction.

Gary J. Algozzine
Robert Algozzine
Deborah J. Lilly

Contents

Sources

Sources

Aehlert B: *ACLS quick review study guide,* ed 2, St Louis, 2001, Mosby.

American Heart Association in Collaboration with the International Liaison Committee on Resuscitation (ILCOR): Part 6: Advanced cardiovascular life support; Section 7: Algorithm approach to ACLS emergencies, *Circulation* 102(suppl I):1-136-171, 2000.

American Society of Health System Pharmacists: *American hospital formulary service,* Bethesda, Md, 2004, The Society.

Bergquist PA: Stability and compatibility of tirofiban hydrochloride during simulated Y-site administration with other drugs, *Am J Health Syst Pharm* 58:1218-1223, 2001.

Gahart BL, Nazareno AR: *2004 intravenous medications,* ed 20, St Louis, 2004, Mosby.

Hazinski MF, Cummins RO, Field JM, editors: *Handbook of emergency cardiovascular care for healthcare providers,* Dallas, 2000, American Heart Association.

Lacy CF, Armstrong LL, Goldman MP, Lance LL: *2003-2004 Drug information handbook,* ed 11, Cleveland, 2003, Lexi-Comp Inc and American Pharmaceutical Association.

Lester RM, Dente-Cassidy AM: *IV medications for critical care,* ed 2, Philadelphia, 1996, WB Saunders.

Medical Economics Staff: *Physician's desk reference 2004,* ed 55, Oradell, NJ, 2000, Medical Economics Company.

Trissel LA: *Handbook of injectable drugs,* ed 12, Bethesda, Md, 2003, American Society of Health System Pharmacists.

Drug Calculation Formulae

Drug Calculation Formulae

1. *Calculate concentration of any drug in a bag (or bottle).*

$$\frac{\text{Amount of drug in bag (mg)}}{\text{Total volume of the bag (mL)}} = \text{Concentration in mg/mL}$$

Example:

$$\frac{\text{Nitroglycerin 25 mg}}{\text{D5W 250 mL}} = 0.1 \text{ mg/mL} = 100 \text{ mcg/mL}$$

2. *Calculate dose administered for a given infusion rate.*

$$\frac{\text{Concentration in bag (mg/mL)} \times \text{infusion rate}}{60 \text{ min}} = \text{Dose per minute}$$

Example: Procainamide 4 mg/mL is infusing at 30 mL/hr. What dose is infusing (mg/min)?

$$\frac{\text{Procainamide 4 mg/mL} \times 30 \text{ mL/hr}}{60 \text{ min}} = 2 \text{ mg/min}$$

3. *Calculate infusion rate for a given dose in mcg/kg/min.*

$$\frac{\text{Body weight (kg)} \times \text{Dose (mcg/kg/min)}}{\text{Drug concentration (mcg/mL)}} = \text{Infusion rate in mL/min} \times 60 \text{ min/hr} = \text{Rate (mL/hr)}$$

Example: Dobutamine 5 mcg/kg/min for a 60-kg patient.

$$\frac{60 \text{ kg} \times 5 \text{ mcg/kg/min}}{2000 \text{ mcg/mL bag}} = 0.15 \text{ mL/min} \times 60 \text{ min/hr} = 9 \text{ mL/hr}$$

4. *Calculation factors (CF).*

$$\frac{\text{Dose (mcg/kg/min)}}{\text{Infusion rate (mL/hr)}} = CF$$

Example: Dobutamine at 5 mcg/kg/min in a 60-kg patient is infusing at 9 mL/hr.

$$\frac{5 \text{ mcg/kg/min}}{9 \text{ mL/hr}} = 0.556 \text{ CF}$$

Calculation factors can be used to quickly convert a particular dose of a drug or infusion to a specific infusion rate in mL/hr or vice versa. This can be helpful when titrating various drugs to effect, and frequent changes in infusion rate may need to be converted to the actual dose of drug administered. For example, if we needed to change the infusion rate from 9 mL/hr of dobutamine to 15 mL/hr to maintain blood pressure, how many mcg/kg/min would be infusing? Multiply the CF by the new rate to get the new dose, or $0.556 \times 15 = 8.34$ mcg/kg/min.

Drug Calculation Formulae

Drug Calculation Formulae

TABLE OF COMMON METRIC CONVERSIONS

1000 micrograms (mcg)	=	1 milligram (mg)
1000 milligrams (mg)	=	1 gram (g)
1000 grams (g)	=	1 kilogram (kg)
1 milliliter (mL)	=	1 cubic centimeter (cc)
1000 milliliters (mL)	=	1 liter (l)

Critical Care Intravenous Infusion Drugs— Quick Mixing Guide

Critical Care Intravenous Infusion Drugs—Quick Mixing Guide

ABCIXIMAB (REOPRO)
Bolus dose: Given IV push
Maintenance dose: Add required maintenance dose to 250 mL D5W

ALTEPLASE (ACTIVASE)
Add 100 mg alteplase to 100 mL sterile water or 50 mg alteplase to 50 mL sterile water
Final concentration: 1 mg/mL

AMINOPHYLLINE (THEOPHYLLINE) 500 MG IN 500 ML D5W
Premade solution
Theophylline 400 mg/500 mL or 800 mg/1000 mL
Final concentration: 1 mg/mL of aminophylline

AMIODARONE (CORDARONE)
Bolus dose: Add 150 mg to 100 mL D5W
Maintenance dose: Add 900 mg to 500 mL D5W in glass bottle
Final concentration: 1.8 mg/mL

ARGATROBAN (ACOVA) 250 MG IN 250 ML NS
Add 250 mg (2.5 mL) argatroban to 250 mL NS
Final concentration: 250 mg/250 mL (1 mg/mL)

ATRACURIUM (TRACRIUM) 250 MG (25 ML) IN 250 ML D5W
Add 250 mg (25 mL) atracurium to 200 mL D5W
Final concentration: 1 mg/mL

BIVALIRUDIN (ANGIOMAX) 250 MG (5 ML) IN 50 ML D5W
Add 250 mg (5 mL) bivalirudin to 50 mL D5W
Final concentration: 5 mg/mL

CISATRACURIUM (NIMBEX) 250 MG IN 250 ML D5W
Add 250 mg (25 × 5-mL vials) cisatracurium to 125 mL D5W
Final concentration: 1 mg/mL

DEXMEDETOMIDINE (PRECEDEX) 2 MG IN 50 ML NS

Add 2 mL Precedex to 48-mL NS minibag
Final concentration: 4 mcg/mL

DILTIAZEM (CARDIZEM) 125 MG IN 100 ML D5W

Add 125 mg (5 × 25-mg vials) diltiazem to 100 mL
   D5W or NS
Final concentration: 125 mg/125 mL (1 mg/mL)

DOBUTAMINE (DOBUTREX) 500 MG IN 250 ML D5W

Premade solution
Final concentration: 500 mg/250 mL (2 mg/mL)

DOPAMINE (INTROPIN) 400 MG IN 250 ML D5W

Premade solution
Final concentration: 400 mg/250 mL (1600 mcg/mL)

DROTRECOGIN ALFA (XIGRIS) (2 × 5 MG) 10 MG IN 100 ML NS

Add 10 mg (2 × 5 mg vials) to 100 mL NS
Final concentration: 10,000 mcg/100 mL (100 mcg/mL)

EPINEPHRINE (ADRENALIN) 1 MG IN 250 ML D5W OR NS

Add 1 mg (1 ampule) epinephrine to 250 mL D5W or NS
Final concentration: 1 mg/250 mL (4 mcg/mL)

EPTIFIBATIDE (INTEGRILIN) 75 MG IN 100-ML VIAL

Premade solution
Bolus dose: From 10-mL vial
Maintenance dose: From 75-mg/100-mL vial

Critical Care Intravenous Infusion Drugs—Quick Mixing Guide

ESMOLOL (BREVIBLOC) 2.5 G IN 250 ML D5W OR NS

Add 2.5 g (10 mL of 250-mg/mL vial) esmolol to 250 mL D5W or NS
Final concentration: 10 mg/mL

FENOLDOPAM (CORLOPAM) 10 MG IN 250 ML D5W OR NS

Add 10 mg (1 mL) fenoldopam to 250 mL D5W or NS
Final concentration: 40 mcg/mL

HALOPERIDOL (HALDOL) FOR RAPID TRANQUILIZATION

Available as 5-mg/mL vial for IV push

HEPARIN 25,000 UNITS IN 500 ML D5W

Premade solution
Final concentration: 25,000 units/500 mL
(50 units/mL)

IBUTILIDE (CORVERT) 1 MG IN 50 ML D5W OR NS

Add 1 mg (10-mL vial) ibutilide to 50 mL D5W or NS
May also be given IV push over 10 minutes

IMMUNE GLOBULIN DOSES

See dosing chart

INAMRINONE (INOCOR) 500 MG IN 100 ML NS

Add 500 mg (5 × 100-mg ampules) inamrinone to 100 mL NS
Final concentration: 500 mg/200 mL (2.5 mg/mL)

INFLIXIMAB (REMICADE) 100 MG TO 900 MG IN 250 ML NS

Add 100 mg to 600 mg (calculate correct dose by weight in dosing charts) to total volume of 250 mL NS
Final concentration: 0.4 to 4 mg/mL.

INSULIN 100 UNITS IN 250 ML NS
Add 100 units (1 mL) insulin to 250 mL NS
Final concentration: 100 units/250 mL (2 units/5 mL)

ISOPROTERENOL (ISUPREL) 1 MG IN 250 ML D5W
Add 1 mg (1 ampule) isoproterenol to 250 mL D5W
Final concentration: 1 mg/250 mL (4 mcg/mL)

LABETALOL (TRANDATE) 200 MG IN 200 ML NS
Add 200 mg (40 mL) labetalol to 160 mL NS
Final concentration: 200 mg/200 mL (1 mg/mL)

LEPIRUDIN (REFLUDAN) 100 MG IN 250 ML NS
Add 100 mg (2 mL) lepirudin to 250 mL NS
Final concentration: 0.4 mg/mL

LIDOCAINE 2 G IN 500 ML D5W
Premade solution
Final concentration: 2 g/500 mL (4 mg/mL)

LORAZEPAM (ATIVAN) 40 MG IN 500 ML D5W
Add 40 mg (10 mL) lorazepam to 500 mL D5W in glass bottle
Final concentration: 0.08 mg/mL

MIDAZOLAM (VERSED) 125 MG IN 125 ML NS
Add 125 mg (25 mL of 5 mg/mL vials) midazolam to 100 mL NS
Final concentration: 1.0 mg/mL

MILRINONE (PRIMACOR) 20 MG IN 100 ML D5W
Premade solution
Final concentration: 0.2 mg/mL

NESIRITIDE (NATRECOR) 1.5 MG IN 250 ML D5W
Add 1.5 mg (5 mL) nesiritide to 250 mL D5W
Final concentration: 1.5 mg/250 mL (6 mcg/mL)

Critical Care Intravenous Infusion Drugs—Quick Mixing Guide

NITROGLYCERIN 25 MG IN 250 ML D5W
Premade solution
Final concentration: 25 mg/250 mL (100 mcg/mL)

NITROPRUSSIDE (NIPRIDE) 50 MG IN 500 ML D5W
Add 50 mg (1 vial) nitroprusside to 500 mL D5W
Final concentration: 50 mg/500 mL (100 mcg/mL)

NOREPINEPHRINE (LEVOPHED) 4 MG IN 250 ML D5W OR NS WITH REGITINE 5 MG/250 ML
Add 4 mg (1 × 4-mg ampule) norepinephrine to 250 mL D5W or NS and add 5 mg Regitine (1 × 5-mg vial) to each 250-mL bag
Final concentration: norepinephrine 4 mg/250 mL (16 mcg/mL)

OCTREOTIDE (SANDOSTATIN) 1200 MCG IN 250 ML D5W OR NS
Add 1200 mcg (2.4 mL) Sandostatin to 250 mL D5W or NS
Final concentration: Sandostatin 4.8 mcg/mL

PANTOPRAZOLE (PROTONIX) 40–80 MG IN 100 ML D5W OR NS
Add 10 mL NS to each 40-mg vial and add contents to 90 mL NS
Final concentration: 40 mg/100 mL (0.4 mg/mL) or 80 mg/100 mL (0.8 mg/mL)

PHENYLEPHRINE (NEO-SYNEPHRINE) 10 MG IN 250 ML D5W
Add 10 mg (1 ampule) phenylephrine to 250 mL D5W
Final concentration: 10 mg/250 mL (40 mcg/mL)

PROCAINAMIDE (PRONESTYL) 1 G IN 250 ML D5W OR NS

Add 1 g (1 vial) Pronestyl to 250 mL D5W or NS

Final concentration: 1 g/250 mL (4 mg/mL)

PROPOFOL (DIPRIVAN) 500 MG/50 ML OR 1 G/100 ML EMULSION

Premade solution

Final concentration: 10 mg/mL

RETEPLASE (RETAVASE) 20-UNIT KIT

Add 10 mL sterile water to 10 units Retavase with kit provided

Repeat for second 10-unit dose

TENECTEPLASE (TNKase)

Add 10 mL sterile water to 50 mg TNKase

Final concentration: 5 mg/mL

TIROFIBAN (AGGRASTAT) 12.5 MG IN 250 ML D5W OR NS

Add 50 mL (12.5 mg) tirofiban to 200 mL D5W or NS

Alternately, add 25 mL (6.25 mg) tirofiban to 100 mL D5W or NS

Final concentration: 50 mcg/mL

Premade 250- and 500-mL bags also available

VASOPRESSIN (PITRESSIN SYNTHETIC) 250 UNITS IN 250 ML

Add 250 units (12.5 mL of 20 units/mL) vasopressin to 250 mL D5W or NS

Final concentration: 250 units/250 mL (1 unit/mL)

Quick Reference Infusion Drug Compatibility and Incompatibility Chart

Drug	Compatibility		Incompatibility	
Abciximab	Unknown or no information		*Unknown or no information*	
Alteplase	Dextrose 5% Lidocaine	Metoprolol Propranolol	*Dobutamine*	*Dopamine*
Aminophylline	Allopurinol Amphotericin B Bretylium Ceftazidime Cimetidine Cladribine Diltiazem Dopamine Doxorubicin Enalaprilat Esmolol Etoposide Famotidine Filgrastim Fluconazole	Foscarnet Gatifloxacin Gemcitabine Granisetron Heparin Inamrinone (Inocor) Labetalol Lidocaine Linezolid Meropenem Morphine Nitroglycerin Paclitaxel Pancuronium Piperacillin	*Amiodarone* *Atracurium* *Chlorpromazine* *(Thorazine)* *Ciprofloxacin* *Clindamycin* *Codeine* *Dobutamine* *Hydralazine* *Hydroxyzine (Vistaril)* *Insulin* *Isoproterenol*	*Meperidine* *(Demerol)* *Norepinephrine* *Ondansetron* *(Zofran)* *Prochlorperazine* *(Compazine)* *Phenytoin (Dilantin)* *Promethazine* *(Phenergan)* *Verapamil*

	Potassium chloride Propofol Ranitidine Remifentanil	Sargramostim Tacrolimus Vecuronium		
Amiodarone	Amikacin Bretylium Clindamycin Dobutamine Dopamine Doxycycline Erythromycin Esmolol Gentamicin Insulin Isoproterenol Labetalol Lidocaine	Metaraminol Metronidazole Midazolam Morphine Nitroglycerin Norepinephrine Penicillin G Phentolamine Phenylephrine Potassium chloride Procainamide Tobramycin Vancomycin	*Aminophylline* *Cefazolin*	*Heparin* *Sodium bicarbonate*
Argatroban	Unknown or no information		*Unknown or no information*	

Continued

Quick Reference Infusion Drug Compatibility and Incompatibility Chart—cont'd

Drug	Compatibility		Incompatibility	
Atracurium	Bretylium Cefazolin Cefuroxime Cimetidine Dobutamine Dopamine Epinephrine Esmolol Etomidate Fentanyl Gentamicin Heparin Hydrocortisone	Isoproterenol Lidocaine Lorazepam Midazolam Milrinone Morphine Nitroglycerin Procainamide Ranitidine Sodium nitroprusside Trimethoprim/sulfa Vancomycin	*Aminophylline* *Diazepam*	*Propofol* *Thiopental*
Bivalirudin	Dexamethasone Digoxin Diphenhydramine Dobutamine Dopamine	Epinephrine Eptifibatide Esmolol Furosemide Heparin	*[including Y-site]* *Alteplase (tPA)* *Amiodarone* *hydrochloride* *Amphotericin B*	*Chlorpromazine* *hydrochloride* *Diazepam* *Prochlorperazine* *Reteplase (rtPA)*

			Streptokinase	Vancomycin hydrochloride
	Hydrocortisone Lidocaine Meperidine Methylprednisolone Midazolam Morphine	Nitroglycerin Potassium chloride Sodium bicarbonate Tirofiban Verapamil		
Cisatracurium	[via Y-site] Alfentanil Amikacin Inamrinone Aztreonam Bretylium Bumetanide Buprenorphine Butorphanol Calcium gluconate Ceftriaxone Chlorpromazine Cimetidine Ciprofloxacin	Clindamycin Dexamethasone Digoxin Diphenhydramine Dobutamine Dopamine Doxycycline Droperidol Enalaprilat Epinephrine Esmolol Famotidine Fentanyl Fluconazole	*Acyclovir* *Aminophylline* *Amphotericin B* *Ampicillin* *Ampicillin/* * sulbactam* *Cefazolin* *Cefotaxime* *Cefotetan* *Cefoxitin* *Ceftazidime* *Cefuroxime* *Diazepam*	*Diprivan* *Furosemide* *Ganciclovir* *Heparin* *Ketorolac* *Methylprednisolone* *Nitroprusside* *Piperacillin* *Thiopental* *Ticarcillin/clavulanate* *Trimethoprim/sulfa* *Zosyn*

Continued

Drug	Compatibility		Incompatibility
	Gatifloxacin	Morphine	
	Gentamicin	Nalbuphine	
	Haloperidol	Nitroglycerin	
	Hydrocortisone	Norepinephrine	
	Hydromorphone	Ofloxacin	
	Hydroxyzine	Ondansetron	
	Imipenem/cilastatin	Phenylephrine	
	Isoproterenol	Potassium chloride	
	Ketorolac	Procainamide	
	Lidocaine	Prochlorperazine	
	Linezolid	Promethazine	
	Lorazepam	Ranitidine	
	Magnesium sulfate	Remifentanil	
	Mannitol	Sufentanil	
	Meperidine	Theophylline	
	Metoclopramide	Ticarcillin	
	Metronidazole	Tobramycin	
	Midazolam	Vancomycin	
	Minocycline	Zidovudine	

Dexmedetomidine	Atracurium besylate	20% Mannitol	*Blood: serum or plasma*	
	Atropine sulfate	Midazolam		
	Fentanyl citrate	Mivacurium chloride		
	Glycopyrrolate	Morphine sulfate		
	bromide	Normal saline		
Diltiazem	Aminophylline	Digoxin	*Acetazolamide*	*Lasix*
	Albumin	Dobutamine	*Acyclovir*	*Methylprednisolone*
	Amikacin	Dopamine	*Aminophylline*	*Phenytoin*
	Amphotericin B	Doxycycline	*Ampicillin*	*Procainamide*
	Aztreonam	Epinephrine	*Diazepam*	*Rifampin*
	Bretylium	Erythromycin	*Hydrocortisone*	*Sodium bicarbonate*
	Bumetanide	Esmolol	*Insulin*	*Thiopental*
	Cefazolin	Fentanyl		
	Cefotaxime	Fluconazole		
	Cefoxitin	Gentamicin		
	Ceftazidime	Heparin		
	Ceftriaxone	Hetastarch		
	Cefuroxime	Hydromorphone		
	Cimetidine	Imipenem/cilastatin		
	Ciprofloxacin	Insulin		
	Clindamycin	Labetalol		

Continued

Drug	Compatibility		Incompatibility	
	Lidocaine	Piperacillin		
	Lorazepam	Potassium chloride		
	Meperidine	Potassium phosphate		
	Metoclopramide	Ranitidine		
	Metronidazole	Nitroglycerin		
	Midazolam	Nitroprusside		
	Milrinone	Norepinephrine		
	Morphine	Theophylline		
	Multivitamins	Ticarcillin/clavulanate		
	Nicardipine	Tobramycin		
	Oxacillin	Trimethoprim/sulfa		
	Penicillin G	Vancomycin		
	Pentamidine	Vecuronium		
Dobutamine	Amiodarone	Calcium chloride	*Acyclovir*	*Cefazolin*
	Atracurium	Calcium gluconate	*Alteplase*	*Cefepime*
	Aztreonam	Ciprofloxacin	*Aminophylline*	*Diazepam*
	Bretylium	Cisatracurium	*Amphotericin B*	*Digoxin*
	Cladribine	Diazepam	*Calcium*	*Foscarnet*

Diltiazem
Docetaxel
Dopamine
Doxorubicin
Enalaprilat
Epinephrine
Etoposide
Famotidine
Fentanyl
Fluconazole
Gatifloxacin
Gemcitabine
Granisetron
Haloperidol
Hydromorphone
Inamrinone
Insulin
Isoproterenol
Labetalol
Levofloxacin

Lidocaine
Linezolid
Lorazepam
Magnesium sulfate
Meperidine
Milrinone
Morphine
Nicardipine
Nitroglycerin
Nitroprusside
Norepinephrine
Pancuronium
Potassium chloride
Procainamide
Propofol
Ranitidine
Remifentanil
Streptokinase
Tacrolimus
Theophylline

Furosemide
Heparin
Hydrocortisone
Indomethacin
Insulin
Magnesium sulfate

Midazolam
Phenytoin
Piperacillin/
tazobactam
Sodium bicarbonate
Thiopental

Continued

Critical Care Intravenous Infusion Drugs—Quick Mixing Guide

Quick Reference Infusion Drug Compatibility and Incompatibility Chart—cont'd

Drug	Compatibility		Incompatibility	
	Thiotepa	Verapamil		
	Tolazoline	Zidovudine		
	Vecuronium			
Dopamine	Alatrofloxacin	Doxorubicin	Acyclovir	Indomethacin
	Aldesleukin	Enalaprilat	Alteplase	Insulin
	Amifostine	Epinephrine	Amphotericin B	Metronidazole
	Aminophylline	Esmolol	Ampicillin	Penicillin G
	Amiodarone	Etoposide	Cefazolin	Potassium
	Atracurium	Famotidine	Cefepime	Sodium bicarbonate
	Aztreonam	Fentanyl	Gentamicin	Thiopental
	Bretylium	Gatifloxacin	Iron dextran	
	Cefpirome	Gemcitabine		
	Ciprofloxacin	Granisetron		
	Cisatracurium	Haloperidol		
	Cladribine	Heparin		
	Diltiazem	Hydrocortisone		
	Dobutamine	Hydromorphone		
	Docetaxel	Inamrinone		

	Labetalol	Pancuronium
	Levofloxacin	Piperacillin/ tazobactam
	Lidocaine	Potassium chloride
	Linezolid	Propofol
	Lorazepam	Ranitidine
	Meperidine	Streptokinase
	Methylprednisolone	Tacrolimus
	Metronidazole	Theophylline
	Midazolam	Vecuronium
	Milrinone	Verapamil
	Nitroglycerin	Warfarin
	Nitroprusside	Zidovudine
	Norepinephrine	
	Ondansetron	
Drotrecogin	Normal saline (NS) Lactated Ringer's (LR) 5% Dextrose in water (D5W) 5% Dextrose in normal saline (D5NS)	*Unknown*

Continued

Quick Reference Infusion Drug Compatibility and Incompatibility Chart—cont'd

Drug	Compatibility		Incompatibility
Epinephrine	Atracurium Diltiazem Dobutamine Dopamine Etomidate Heparin Inamrinone	Labetalol Midazolam Nitroglycerin Norepinephrine Potassium chloride Propofol	*Aminophylline* *Sodium bicarbonate* *Thiopental*
Eptifibatide	Alteplase (tPA) Atropine D5NS Dobutamine	Heparin Lidocaine Meperidine Metoprolol	*Furosemide*

	Midazolam Morphine Nitroglycerin Normal saline	Potassium chloride (up to 60 mEq) Verapamil	
Esmolol	Amikacin Aminophylline Amiodarone Ampicillin Atracurium Bretylium Butorphanol Calcium chloride Cefazolin Ceftazidime Chloramphenicol Cimetidine Cisatracurium Clindamycin Diltiazem Dopamine Enalaprilat	Erythromycin Famotidine Fentanyl Gatifloxacin Gentamicin Heparin Hydrocortisone Insulin Labetalol Linezolid Magnesium sulfate Methyldopa Metronidazole Midazolam Morphine Nafcillin Nitroglycerin	*Amphotericin B* *Furosemide* *Warfarin*

Continued

Drug	Compatibility		Incompatibility
	Nitroprusside Norepinephrine Pancuronium Penicillin G Phenytoin Piperacillin Polymyxin B Potassium chloride Potassium phosphate	Propofol Ranitidine Remifentanil Sodium acetate Streptomycin Tacrolimus Trimethoprim/sulfa Vancomycin Vecuronium	
Fenoldopam	[In-line compatibility] Cefazolin, dopamine, epinephrine, gentamicin, heparin, lidocaine, and nitroprusside		[In-line incompatibility] *Alkaline solutions* *Furosemide*
Haloperidol	Dobutamine Dopamine Lidocaine	Midazolam Nitroglycerin Theophylline	*Heparin* *Nitroprusside* *Procainamide*

Heparin	Acyclovir	Cladribine	*Alatrofloxacin*	*Ergotamine*
	Aldesleukin	Clindamycin	*Alteplase*	*Filgrastim*
	Allopurinol	Cyanocobalamin	*Amikacin*	*Gatifloxacin*
	Amifostine	Cyclophosphamide	*Amiodarone*	*Gentamicin*
	Aminophylline	Cytarabine	*Amphotericin B*	*Haloperidol*
	Ampicillin	Dexamethasone	*Amsacrine*	*Levofloxacin*
	Ampicillin/sulbactam	Digoxin	*Ciprofloxacin*	*Methadone*
	Atracurium	Diltiazem	*Codeine phosphate*	*Nicardipine*
	Atropine	Diphenhydramine	*Diazepam*	*Phenergan*
	Aztreonam	Docetaxel	*Dilantin*	*Tobramycin*
	Betamethasone	Dopamine	*Dobutamine*	*Vancomycin*
	Bleomycin	Doxorubicin	*Doxycycline*	
	Calcium gluconate	Edrophonium		
	Cefazolin	Enalaprilat		
	Cefotetan	Epinephrine		
	Ceftazidime	Erythromycin		
	Ceftriaxone	Esmolol		
	Chlordiazepoxide	Ethacrynate		
	Chlorpromazine	Etoposide		
	Cimetidine	Famotidine		
	Cisplatin	Fentanyl		

Continued

Quick Reference Infusion Drug Compatibility and Incompatibility Chart—cont'd

Drug	Compatibility		Incompatibility
	Fluconazole	Meropenem	
	Fludarabine	Methotrexate	
	Fluorouracil	Methyldopa	
	Foscarnet	Metoclopramide	
	Furosemide	Metronidazole	
	Gemcitabine	Midazolam	
	Granisetron	Milrinone	
	Hydralazine	Minocycline	
	Hydrocortisone	Mitomycin	
	Hydromorphone	Morphine	
	Isoproterenol	Nafcillin	
	Insulin	Neostigmine	
	Kanamycin	Nitroglycerin	
	Leucovorin	Nitroprusside	
	Lidocaine	Norepinephrine	
	Linezolid	Ondansetron	
	Lorazepam	Oxacillin	
	Magnesium sulfate	Oxytocin	
	Meperidine	Paclitaxel	

	Pancuronium Penicillin G Pentazocine Piperacillin Potassium chloride Procainamide	Prochlorperazine Theophylline Vinblastine Vincristine Zidovudine	
Ibutilide		*Avoid use with other antiarrhythmic agents (disopyramide, quinidine, and procainamide) due to increased toxicity. Also, amiodarone and sotalol should be avoided due to their potential to prolong refractoriness.* *Avoid use with phenothiazines, tricyclic and tetracyclic antidepressants, and nonsedating Antihistamines (terfenadine [Seldane] and astemizole [Hismanal]) due to QT prolongation.*
Immune Globulin Intravenous	None. Administer via a separate IV line with no other medications.	*Unknown*

Continued

Quick Reference Infusion Drug Compatibility and Incompatibility Chart—cont'd

Drug	Compatibility		Incompatibility	
Inamrinone	Aminophylline Atropine Bretylium Calcium chloride Cimetidine Cisatracurium Digoxin Dobutamine Dopamine Epinephrine Famotidine	Hydrocortisone Isoproterenol Lidocaine Methylprednisolone Nitroglycerin Nitroprusside Norepinephrine Phenylephrine Potassium chloride Propofol	*Dextrose solutions* *Furosemide (Lasix)*	*Procainamide* *Sodium bicarbonate*
Infliximab	Unknown or no information		*Unknown or no information*	
Insulin Drip	Amiodarone Ampicillin Ampicillin/sulbactam Aztreonam Bretylium Cefazolin	Cefotetan Cimetidine Clarithromycin Diltiazem Dobutamine Esmolol	*Aminophylline* *Bretylium* *Chlorothiazide* *Cytarabine* *Dobutamine* *Dopamine*	*Labetalol* *Levofloxacin* *Lidocaine* *Methylprednisolone* *Nafcillin* *Norepinephrine*

	Compatible		Incompatible	
	Famotidine Gentamicin Heparin Imipenem/cilastatin Indomethacin Lidocaine Magnesium sulfate Meperidine Meropenem Midazolam Milrinone Morphine	Nitroglycerin Nitroprusside Oxytocin Pentobarbital Potassium chloride Propofol Ritodrine Sodium bicarbonate Tacrolimus Terbutaline Ticarcillin/clavulanate Verapamil	*Octreotide* *Pentobarbital* *Phenytoin* *Ranitidine*	*Secobarbital* *Sodium bicarbonate* *Thiopental*
Isoproterenol	Amiodarone Atracurium Bretylium Calcium chloride Cimetidine Cisatracurium Dobutamine Dopamine Famotidine	Floxacillin Heparin Hydrocortisone Inamrinone Levofloxacin Magnesium sulfate Milrinone Multivitamins Pancuronium	*Alkaline solutions* *Aminophylline* *Furosemide*	*Lidocaine* *Sodium bicarbonate*

Continued

Drug	Compatibility		Incompatibility
	Potassium chloride Propofol Ranitidine Remifentanil Sodium succinate Succinylcholine	Tacrolimus Vecuronium Verapamil Vitamin B complex with C	
Labetalol	Amikacin Aminophylline Amiodarone Ampicillin Butorphanol Calcium gluconate Cefazolin Ceftazidime Cimetidine Clindamycin Chloramphenicol Diltiazem Dobutamine	Dopamine Enalaprilat Epinephrine Erythromycin Esmolol Famotidine Fentanyl Gatifloxacin Gentamicin Heparin Hydromorphone Lidocaine Linezolid	*Amphotericin B* *Nafcillin* *Ceftriaxone* *Sodium bicarbonate* *Furosemide* *Thiopental* *Heparin* *Warfarin* *Insulin*

	Lorazepam Magnesium sulfate Meperidine Metronidazole Midazolam Milrinone Morphine Nicardipine Nitroglycerin Nitroprusside Norepinephrine	Oxacillin Penicillin G Piperacillin Potassium chloride Propofol Ranitidine Tobramycin Trimethoprim/sulfa Vancomycin Vecuronium	
Lepirudin	Unknown or no information		*Unknown or no information*
Lidocaine	Alteplase Aminophylline Amiodarone Atracurium Bretylium Bupivacaine Calcium chloride Calcium gluconate	Cefazolin Chloramphenicol Chlorothiazide Cimetidine Ciprofloxacin Cisatracurium Clarithromycin Clonidine	*Amphotericin B* *Ampicillin* *Cefazolin* *Ceftriaxone* *Dacarbazine* *Epinephrine*	*Isoproterenol* *Methohexital* *Norepinephrine* *Phenytoin* *Sodium bicarbonate*

Continued

Drug	Compatibility		Incompatibility
	Dexamethasone	Hydroxyzine	
	Digoxin	Inamrinone	
	Diltiazem	Insulin	
	Diphenhydramine	Ketamine	
	Dobutamine	Labetalol	
	Dopamine	Levofloxacin	
	Enalaprilat	Linezolid	
	Ephedrine	Meperidine	
	Erythromycin	Mephentermine	
	Etomidate	Metoclopramide	
	Famotidine	Milrinone	
	Fentanyl	Morphine	
	Floxacillin	Nafcillin	
	Flumazenil	Nitroglycerin	
	Furosemide	Nitroprusside	
	Gatifloxacin	Penicillin G	
	Glycopyrrolate	Pentobarbital	
	Haloperidol	Phenylephrine	
	Heparin	Potassium chloride	
	Hydrocortisone	Procainamide	

	Promazine	Streptokinase	
	Propafenone	Tetracaine	
	Propofol	Theophylline	
	Ranitidine	Tirofiban	
	Sodium bicarbonate	Verapamil	
	Sodium phosphate		
Lorazepam	Acyclovir	Clonidine	*Aldesleukin*	*Idarubicin*
	Albumin	Cyclophosphamide	*Atracurium*	*Imipenem/cilastatin*
	Allopurinol	Cytarabine	*Aztreonam*	*Ranitidine*
	Amifostine	Dexamethasone	*Buprenorphine*	*Sargramostim*
	Amikacin	Diltiazem	*Dexamethasone*	*Sufentanil*
	Amphotericin B	Dobutamine	*Floxacillin*	*Thiopental*
	Atracurium	Docetaxel	*Foscarnet*	*Zofran*
	Bumetanide	Dopamine		
	Cefepime	Doxorubicin		
	Cefotaxime	Epinephrine		
	Cimetidine	Erythromycin		
	Ciprofloxacin	Etomidate		
	Cisatracurium	Etoposide		
	Cisplatin	Famotidine		
	Cladribine	Fentanyl		

Continued

Quick Reference Infusion Drug Compatibility and Incompatibility Chart—cont'd

Drug	Compatibility		Incompatibility
	Filgrastim	Milrinone	
	Fluconazole	Morphine	
	Fludarabine	Nicardipine	
	Fosphenytoin	Nitroglycerin	
	Furosemide	Norepinephrine	
	Gatifloxacin	Paclitaxel	
	Gemcitabine	Pancuronium	
	Gentamicin	Piperacillin	
	Granisetron	Piperacillin/tazobactam	
	Haloperidol	Potassium chloride	
	Heparin	Propofol	
	Hydrocortisone	Ranitidine	
	Hydromorphone	Tacrolimus	
	Labetalol	Teniposide	
	Levofloxacin	Thiotepa	
	Linezolid	Vancomycin	
	Methotrexate	Vecuronium	
	Metronidazole	Vinorelbine	
	Midazolam	Zidovudine	

Midazolam

Compatible		Incompatible (italic)	
Amiodarone	Esmolol	*Albumin*	*Fosphenytoin*
Amikacin	Famotidine	*Amphotericin B*	*Furosemide*
Atracurium	Fentanyl	*Ampicillin*	*Hydrocortisone*
Atropine	Gatifloxacin	*Bumetanide*	*Imipenem/cilastatin*
Buprenorphine	Gentamicin	*Butorphanol*	*Methotrexate*
Butorphanol	Haloperidol	*Ceftazidime*	*Nafcillin*
Calcium gluconate	Heparin	*Cefuroxime*	*Phenobarbital*
Cefazolin	Hydromorphone	*Clonidine*	*Prochlorperazine*
Cefotaxime	Hydroxyzine	*Dexamethasone*	*Propofol*
Chlorpromazine	Insulin	*Dimenhydrinate*	*Ranitidine*
Cimetidine	Labetalol	*Dobutamine*	*Sodium bicarbonate*
Ciprofloxacin	Linezolid	*Floxacillin*	*Thiopental*
Cisatracurium	Lorazepam	*Foscarnet*	*Trimethoprim/sulfa*
Clindamycin	Meperidine		
Digoxin	Methylprednisolone		
Diltiazem	Metoclopramide		
Diphenhydramine	Metronidazole		
Dopamine	Milrinone		
Droperidol	Morphine		
Epinephrine	Nicardipine		
Erythromycin	Nitroglycerin		

Continued

Quick Reference Infusion Drug Compatibility and Incompatibility Chart—cont'd

Drug	Compatibility		Incompatibility
	Nitroprusside Ondansetron Pancuronium Piperacillin Potassium chloride Promethazine	Ranitidine Theophylline Tobramycin Vancomycin Vecuronium	
Milrinone	Atracurium Atropine Calcium chloride Calcium gluconate Cimetidine Digoxin Diltiazem Dobutamine Dopamine Epinephrine Fentanyl Heparin	Hydromorphone Insulin Isoproterenol Labetalol Lidocaine Lorazepam Magnesium sulfate Midazolam Morphine Nicardipine Nitroglycerin Nitroprusside	*Bumetanide* *Furosemide* *Procainamide*

	Norepinephrine Pancuronium Potassium chloride Propofol Propranolol Quinidine gluconate Ranitidine	Sodium bicarbonate Theophylline Thiopental Torsemide Vecuronium Verapamil	

Nesiritide	D5W
	NS
		D5½NS
		D5¼NS
			Bumetanide
			Enalaprilat
			Ethacrynic acid (Ethacrynate)
			Furosemide
			Heparin*
			Hydralazine
			Injectable drugs with the preservative
			  sodium metabisulfite
			Insulin
			
			*Do not administer via heparin-coated
			  central catheter.

Continued

Quick Reference Infusion Drug Compatibility and Incompatibility Chart—cont'd

Drug	Compatibility	Incompatibility
Nitroglycerin	[via Y-site] Amiodarone Amphotericin B Atracurium Cisatracurium Diltiazem Dobutamine Dopamine Epinephrine Esmolol Famotidine Fentanyl Fluconazole Furosemide Gatifloxacin Haloperidol Heparin Hydromorphone Inamrinone Insulin Labetalol Lidocaine Linezolid Lorazepam Midazolam Milrinone Morphine Nicardipine Nitroprusside Norepinephrine Pancuronium Propofol Ranitidine Streptokinase Tacrolimus Theophylline Thiopental Vecuronium Warfarin	*Do not mix nitroglycerin in the same bottle with any other drugs.*

Nitroprusside	Atracurium Cimetidine Diltiazem Dobutamine Dopamine Enalaprilat Esmolol Famotidine Heparin Inamrinone Indomethacin Insulin Labetalol	Lidocaine Midazolam Milrinone Morphine Nitroglycerin Pancuronium Propofol Ranitidine Tacrolimus Theophylline Verapamil Vecuronium	*No other drug should be added to the infusion fluid for simultaneous administration with nitroprusside.*	
Norepinephrine	Amikacin Amiodarone Calcium chloride Calcium gluconate Cimetidine Cisatracurium Corticotropin	Diltiazem Dimenhydrinate Dobutamine Dopamine Epinephrine Esmolol Famotidine	*Aminophylline* *Amobarbital* *Barbiturates* *Cephalothin* *Cephapirin* *Chlorothiazide* *Insulin*	*Nafcillin* *Phenobarbital* *Phenytoin* *Sodium bicarbonate* *Streptomycin* *Thiopental* *Whole blood*

Continued

Drug	Compatibility		Incompatibility
	Fentanyl	Midazolam	
	Furosemide	Milrinone	
	Haloperidol	Morphine	
	Heparin	Multivitamins	
	Hydrocortisone	Nicardipine	
	Hydromorphone	Nitroglycerin	
	Inamrinone	Potassium chloride	
	Labetalol	Propofol	
	Lorazepam	Ranitidine	
	Magnesium sulfate	Remifentanil	
	Meropenem	Succinylcholine	
	Methylprednisolone	Vecuronium	
Octreotide	Heparin		*None specified. Because of lack of data, this drug should not be mixed with other medications except as noted here.*
	Total parenteral nutrition		

Pantoprazole	No known documented. Protonix should not be infused with other drug infusions.		*A single dedicated line is usually preferred. If a Y-site is used, position it closest to the patient. The line should be flushed with D5W, NS, or LR.*
Phenylephrine	Amiodarone Chloramphenicol Cisatracurium Dobutamine Etomidate Famotidine Haloperidol Inamrinone	Levofloxacin Lidocaine Potassium chloride Remifentanil Sodium bicarbonate Zidovudine	*Nitroglycerin Nitroprusside Phenytoin*	*Propofol Thiopental*
Procainamide	Amiodarone Atracurium Cisatracurium Diltiazem Dobutamine Famotidine Flumazenil	Heparin Hydrocortisone Lidocaine Potassium chloride Ranitidine Remifentanil Verapamil	*Aminophylline Barbiturates Bretylium Diltiazem Esmolol Ethacrynate*	*Inamrinone Magnesium sulfate Milrinone Phenytoin Sodium bicarbonate*

Continued

Drug	Compatibility		Incompatibility	
Propofol	Acyclovir	Cisplatin	*Amikacin*	*Methotrexate*
	Alfentanil	Clindamycin	*Amphotericin B*	*Methylprednisolone*
	Aminophylline	Cyclophosphamide	*Ascorbic acid*	*Metoclopramide*
	Ampicillin	Cyclosporine	*Atracurium*	*Midazolam*
	Aztreonam	Cytarabine	*Atropine*	*Minocycline*
	Bumetanide	Dexamethasone	*Blood*	*Mitoxantrone*
	Buprenorphine	Diphenhydramine	*Bretylium*	*Pancuronium*
	Butorphanol	Dobutamine	*Calcium chloride*	*Phenylephrine*
	Calcium gluconate	Dopamine	*Ciprofloxacin*	*Phenytoin*
	Carboplatin	Doxycycline	*Diazepam*	*Plasma*
	Cefazolin	Droperidol	*Digoxin*	*Serum*
	Cefotaxime	Enalaprilat	*Doxacurium*	*Tobramycin*
	Cefotetan	Ephedrine	*Doxorubicin*	*Verapamil*
	Cefotaxime	Epinephrine	*Gentamicin*	
	Ceftazidime	Esmolol		
	Ceftizoxime	Famotidine		
	Ceftriaxone	Fentanyl		
	Cefuroxime	Fluconazole		
	Chlorpromazine	Fluorouracil		
	Cimetidine	Furosemide		

Ganciclovir
Glycopyrrolate
Granisetron
Haloperidol
Heparin
Hydrocortisone
Hydromorphone
Hydroxyzine
Ifosfamide
Imipenem/cilastatin
Inamrinone
Insulin
Isoproterenol
Ketamine
Labetalol
Levorphanol
Lidocaine
Lorazepam
Magnesium sulfate
Mannitol
Meperidine

Midazolam
Milrinone
Morphine
Nafcillin
Nalbuphine
Naloxone
Nitroglycerin
Nitroprusside
Norepinephrine
Ofloxacin
Ondansetron
Paclitaxel
Pentobarbital
Phenobarbital
Phenylephrine
Piperacillin
Potassium chloride
Prochlorperazine
Propranolol
Ranitidine
Scopolamine

Continued

Drug	Compatibility		Incompatibility
	Sodium bicarbonate Succinylcholine Sufentanil Thiopental	Ticarcillin Ticarcillin/clavulanate Vancomycin Vecuronium	
Reteplase	None		*All medications.* *Retavase should be administered in separate IV line whenever possible and should not be mixed with any other medications.*
Tenecteplase	NS		*All dextrose solutions.*
Tirofiban	Atropine Dobutamine Dopamine Epinephrine Famotidine Furosemide Heparin	Lidocaine Midazolam Morphine Nitroglycerin Potassium chloride Propranolol	*Diazepam* *(Valium)*
Vasopressin	Unknown or no information		*Unknown or no information*

Intravenous Infusion Drugs

Abciximab (ReoPro)

USES

1. An adjunct to percutaneous coronary interventions for prevention of cardiac ischemic complications during or after the procedure.
2. Prevention of cardiac ischemia with unstable angina that is not responding to conventional therapy when cardiac intervention is planned within 24 hours.

SOLUTION PREPARATION

Mix the required dose of abciximab per the dosing chart into a 250-mL bag of D5W or NS. Drug must be withdrawn from the vial using a sterile, nonpyrogenic, low protein–binding 0.2, 0.22, or 5 micron filter. Abciximab is supplied in 10-mg/5-mL vials.

DOSE

Usual dose is 0.25 mg/kg IV bolus over 10-60 minutes before intervention. Immediately follow bolus with a 0.125-mcg/kg/min infusion for 12 hours. Maximum dose is 10 mcg/kg/min. See dosing chart.

WARNINGS

1. Increased risk of bleeding, especially in the presence of anticoagulants or thrombolytics.
2. Heparin doses may be reduced during abciximab infusions.
3. Administration is contraindicated in cases of active internal bleeding, a history of GI bleeding within 6 weeks, cardiovascular accident (CVA) within 2 years, thrombocytopenia, or uncontrolled hypertension.
4. Platelet counts, PT, PTT, and ACT should be monitored at regular intervals.

ADVERSE REACTIONS

Bleeding is the major side effect. Major bleeding requiring transfusion has been reported. Intracranial hemorrhage or stroke is possible. Minor bleeding—such as increased bruising, hematuria, and hematemesis—is also possible.

INCOMPATIBILITY

Abciximab should be administered in a separate IV line whenever possible. No incompatibilities have been reported with infusion IV fluids or commonly used cardiovascular medications.

NURSING CONSIDERATIONS

1. Use a separate IV site for administration. An infusion pump or controller should be used. Additional filtration is not required if the infusion bag is prepared using at least a 5-micron filter.
2. Watch closely for bleeding or anaphylaxis.
3. Arterial/venous sheaths may be removed while abciximab is infusing, provided that ACT is adequate and direct pressure is held for 30 minutes.
4. Minimize arterial and venous punctures.
5. Platelets may need to be administered if platelet counts drop below 100,000 or as treatment for active bleeding.

Abciximab (ReoPro)

Weight-Based Dosing Chart for Abciximab (ReoPro)
Initial Bolus and Continuous Infusion (0.125 mcg/kg/min for 12 hours)

Patient weight	Bolus dose (mg) (0.25 mg/kg)	Abciximab to add to NS 250 mL (mg)	Infusion rate (mL/hr)
46 kg	11.50 (5.8 mL)	4.14 (2.1 mL)	21
47 kg	11.75 (5.9 mL)	4.23 (2.1 mL)	21
48 kg	12 (6 mL)	4.32 (2.2 mL)	21
49 kg	12.25 (6.1 mL)	4.41 (2.2 mL)	21
50 kg	12.50 (6.3 mL)	4.50 (2.3 mL)	21
51 kg	12.75 (6.4 mL)	4.59 (2.3 mL)	21
52 kg	13 (6.5 mL)	4.68 (2.3 mL)	21
53 kg	13.25 (6.6 mL)	4.77 (2.4 mL)	21
54 kg	13.50 (6.8 mL)	4.86 (2.4 mL)	21
55 kg	13.75 (6.9 mL)	4.95 (2.5 mL)	21
56 kg	14 (7 mL)	5.04 (2.5 mL)	21
57 kg	14.25 (7.1 mL)	5.13 (2.6 mL)	21
58 kg	14.50 (7.3 mL)	5.22 (2.6 mL)	21
59 kg	14.75 (7.4 mL)	5.31 (2.7 mL)	21
60 kg	15 (7.5 mL)	5.40 (2.7 mL)	21
61 kg	15.25 (7.6 mL)	5.49 (2.7 mL)	21

62 kg	15.50 (7.8 mL)	5.58 (2.8 mL)	21
63 kg	15.75 (7.9 mL)	5.67 (2.8 mL)	21
64 kg	16 (8 mL)	5.76 (2.9 mL)	21
65 kg	16.25 (8.1 mL)	5.85 (2.9 mL)	21
66 kg	16.50 (8.3 mL)	5.94 (3 mL)	21
67 kg	16.75 (8.4 mL)	6.03 (3 mL)	21
68 kg	17 (8.5 mL)	6.12 (3 mL)	21
69 kg	17.25 (8.6 mL)	6.21 (3.1 mL)	21
70 kg	17.50 (8.8 mL)	6.30 (3.1 mL)	21
71 kg	17.75 (8.9 mL)	6.39 (3.2 mL)	21
72 kg	18 (9 mL)	6.48 (3.2 mL)	21
73 kg	18.25 (9.1 mL)	6.57 (3.3 mL)	21
74 kg	18.50 (9.3 mL)	6.66 (3.3 mL)	21
75 kg	18.75 (9.4 mL)	6.75 (3.4 mL)	21
76 kg	19 (9.5 mL)	6.84 (3.4 mL)	21
77 kg	19.25 (9.6 mL)	6.93 (3.5 mL)	21
78 kg	19.50 (9.8 mL)	7.02 (3.5 mL)	21
79 kg	19.75 (9.9 mL)	7.11 (3.6 mL)	21
80 kg	20 (10 mL)	7.20 (3.6 mL)	21
85 kg	21.30 (10.6 mL)	7.20 (3.6 mL)	21
90 kg	22.50 (11.3 mL)	7.20 (3.6 mL)	21

Continued

Abciximab (ReoPro)

Weight-Based Dosing Chart for Abciximab (ReoPro)
Initial Bolus and Continuous Infusion (0.125 mcg/kg/min for 12 hours)

Patient weight	Bolus dose (mg) (0.25 mg/kg)	Abciximab to add to NS 250 mL (mg)	Infusion rate (mL/hr)
95 kg	23.80 (11.9 mL)	7.20 (3.6 mL)	21
100 kg	25 (12.5 mL)	7.20 (3.6 mL)	21
105 kg	26.30 (13.1 mL)	7.20 (3.6 mL)	21
110 kg	27.50 (13.8 mL)	7.20 (3.6 mL)	21
115 kg	28.80 (14.4 mL)	7.20 (3.6 mL)	21

Patients who weigh >80 kg will be infused at a fixed rate of 10 mcg/min (21 mL/hr). Refrigerate and reuse any remaining abciximab within 7 days of initial use of vial. Abciximab is very expensive.

Alteplase (Activase)

USES

1. As a thrombolytic for treatment of acute myocardial infarction (AMI), with chest pain >20 minutes and onset within <12-24 hours, to improve ventricular function.
2. For acute pulmonary embolism (PE), age <75 years and within 5 days of thrombus formation.
3. For acute ischemic stroke, age <75 years and within the first 3 hours of the onset of symptoms.

SOLUTION PREPARATION

Reconstitute 100-mg vial alteplase in 100 mL sterile water. Final concentration: 1 mg/mL.

DOSE

1. *AMI* (front-loaded dose): Give 15 mg (15 mL) bolus, then infuse 0.75 mg/kg over 30 minutes (up to 50 mg), then give 0.5 mg/kg over the next 60 minutes (not more than 35 mg). For patients <67 kg: Give 15-mg bolus IV push, then 0.75 mg/kg over 30 minutes, then 0.5 mg/kg over 60 minutes.
2. *PE:* 100 mg over 2 hours, infuse at 50 mL/hr.
3. *Stroke:* 0.9 mg/kg (up to 90 mg). Infuse 10% (0.09 mg/kg) as a bolus dose, followed by the remainder (0.81 mg/kg) as a continuous infusion over 60 minutes. Maximum total dose is 90 mg.

WARNINGS

1. Increased risk of bleeding, especially in the presence of anticoagulation.
2. *For AMI patients:* Heparin doses of 5000-unit bolus and 1000 units/hr or 800 units/hr for patients <80 kg may be used. *For stroke patients:* Start heparin infusion without loading bolus doses.
3. Administration of alteplase is contraindicated in cases of active internal bleeding, history of GI bleeding within 6 weeks, trauma or surgery within 1 month, thrombocytopenia, uncontrolled hypertension (SBP >185, DBP >110, unresponsive to nitrates or calcium antagonists) intracranial neoplasm, arteriovenous malformations, or aneurysm. Also contraindicated with history of

cerebrovascular accident (CVA) within 1 month, seizure occurring at the time of stroke, or any suspicion of hemorrhagic stroke.

ADVERSE REACTIONS

1. Bleeding is the major side effect. Intracranial hemorrhage (0.4%-0.87%) or stroke has been reported as a complication. Minor bleeding such as increased bruising, hematuria, GI bleeding, bleeding at the injection site (up to 15.3%), and genitourinary hemorrhage is possible.
2. Allergic reactions and anaphylaxis are rare.
3. Hypotension and arrhythmias are also possible.

INCOMPATIBILITY

Dobutamine   Dopamine

COMPATIBILITY

Dextrose 5%   Metoprolol
Lidocaine   Propranolol

NURSING CONSIDERATIONS

1. Use a separate IV site; do not administer with heparin because of incompatibility.
2. Watch closely for bleeding, particularly within the first hour of administration, or anaphylaxis.
3. Minimize arterial and venous punctures for at least 24 hours after administration.
4. Heparin and aspirin (160-325 mg) should be used with alteplase to reduce to risk of rethrombosis.

Alteplase (Activase)

Alteplase (Activase, t-PA) Dosing Chart—Acute Myocardial Infarction
Alteplase 100 mg Added to 100 mL Sterile Water (Concentration: 1 mg/mL)

Patient weight	Initial loading dose over 1-2 min	Second dose (0.75 mg/kg) over 30 min	Final dose (0.5 mg/kg) over 60 min
50 kg	15 mg	38 mg (75 mL/hr)	25 mg (25 mL/hr)
60 kg	15 mg	45 mg (90 mL/hr)	30 mg (30 mL/hr)
70 kg	15 mg	50 mg (100 mL/hr)	35 mg (35 mL/hr)
80 kg	15 mg	50 mg (100 mL/hr)	35 mg (35 mL/hr)
90 kg	15 mg	50 mg (100 mL/hr)	35 mg (35 mL/hr)

Alteplase (Activase, t-PA) Dosing Chart—Acute Ischemic Stroke
Alteplase 100 mg Added to 100 mL Sterile Water or 50 mg Added to 50 mL Sterile Water (Concentration: 1 mg/mL)

Patient weight	Initial loading dose over 1-2 min (0.09 mg/kg)	Second dose (0.81 mg/kg) over 60 min	Total dose (0.9 mg/kg)
50 kg	4 mg	41 mg (41 mL/hr)	45 mg
60 kg	5 mg	49 mg (49 mL/hr)	54 mg
70 kg	6 mg	57 mg (57 mL/hr)	63 mg
80 kg	7 mg	65 mg (65 mL/hr)	72 mg
90 kg	8 mg	73 mg (73 mL/hr)	81 mg
≥100 kg	9 mg	81 mg (81 mL/hr)	90 mg

Alteplase (Activase)

Aminophylline (Theophylline)

USES

1. Symptomatic relief or prevention of bronchial asthma and reversible bronchospasm associated with chronic bronchitis and emphysema.
2. May significantly improve pulmonary function and dyspnea in patients with chronic obstructive pulmonary disease (COPD).

SOLUTION PREPARATION

Infusions of theophylline 400 mg/500 mL or 800 mg/1000 mL D5W (equivalent to 1 mg/mL aminophylline) are available.

NOTE: Aminophylline IV is equivalent to 80% theophylline; for example, to give aminophylline 30 mg/hr, run standard theophylline solutions at 30 mL/hr, or to give aminophylline 20 mg/hr, run standard theophylline solutions at 20 mL/hr.

DOSE

1. Dosage will vary and depend on patient's condition, concomitant disease state, and prior theophylline use (serum theophylline level).

2. Loading dose
   a. Patients not currently receiving theophylline, give aminophylline 6 mg/kg.
   b. To increase levels in patients currently receiving theophylline, give aminophylline 0.5 mg/kg to increase theophylline level by 1 mcg/mL.
   c. *Goal serum level:* 5-15 mcg/mL.
3. Maintenance infusion
   a. Adjust dose according to serum theophylline levels.
   b. *Usual dosage range:* Aminophylline 0.25-0.75 mg/kg/hr.

WARNINGS

1. *Toxicity warning:* Monitor serum levels to avoid toxicity; normal levels are 5-15 mcg/mL. Incidence of toxicity increases significantly with serum levels >20 mcg/mL, with symptoms including ventricular arrhythmias, convulsions, and death.
2. Patients with decreased ability to clear plasma of aminophylline (e.g., those with impaired liver function, congestive heart failure (CHF), >55 years

of age, sustained high fever) are at increased risk of toxicity.
3. Aminophylline may cause arrhythmia; monitor levels if significant changes in HR or rhythm occur. Ventricular arrhythmias will respond to lidocaine.

ADVERSE REACTIONS

1. Adverse reactions rarely occur when serum levels are <20 mcg/mL.
   a. Serum levels >20 mcg/mL: Nausea, vomiting, diarrhea, headache, insomnia, irritability.
   b. Serum levels >35 mcg/mL: Hyperglycemia, hypotension, cardiac arrhythmias, tachycardia.
2. *CNS:* Irritability, restlessness, headache, insomnia, reflex hyperexcitability, muscle twitching, convulsions.
3. *GI:* Nausea, vomiting, epigastric pain, hematemesis, diarrhea; may induce gastroesophageal reflux.
4. *Cardiovascular:* Palpitations, tachycardia, extrasystoles, hypotension, circulatory failure, ventricular arrhythmias.
5. *Other:* Tachypnea, proteinuria, fever, hyperglycemia, rash.

INCOMPATIBILITY

Amiodarone
Atracurium
Chlorpromazine
 (Thorazine)
Ciprofloxacin
Clindamycin
Codeine
Dobutamine
Hydralazine
Hydroxyzine (Vistaril)
Insulin
Isoproterenol
Meperidine (Demerol)
Norepinephrine
Ondansetron (Zofran)
Prochlorperazine
 (Compazine)
Phenytoin (Dilantin)
Promethazine
 (Phenergan)
Verapamil

COMPATIBILITY

Allopurinol
Amphotericin B
Bretylium
Ceftazidime
Cimetidine
Cladribine
Diltiazem
Dopamine
Doxorubicin
Enalaprilat

Aminophylline (Theophylline)

Esmolol
Etoposide
Famotidine
Filgrastim
Fluconazole
Foscarnet
Gatifloxacin
Gemcitabine
Granisetron
Heparin
Inamrinone (Inocor)
Labetalol
Lidocaine
Linezolid

Meropenem
Morphine
Nitroglycerin
Paclitaxel
Pancuronium
Piperacillin
Potassium chloride
Propofol
Ranitidine
Remifentanil
Sargramostim
Tacrolimus
Vecuronium

NURSING CONSIDERATIONS

1. Consult the Aminophylline Drip Rate Calculation Chart to determine the drip rate.
2. Aminophylline should be administered by an IV pump to ensure controlled infusion.
3. Monitor serum aminophylline levels; call physician if elevated levels are noted. Monitor patients for signs of toxicity.

Aminophylline Drip Rate Calculation Chart
Theophylline 400 mg/500 mL or 800 mg/1000 mL (Aminophylline concentration: 1 mg/mL)

Dose	Infusion rate
10 mg/hr	10 mL/hr
15 mg/hr	15 mL/hr
20 mg/hr	20 mL/hr
25 mg/hr	25 mL/hr
30 mg/hr	30 mL/hr
35 mg/hr	35 mL/hr
40 mg/hr	40 mL/hr
45 mg/hr	45 mL/hr
50 mg/hr	50 mL/hr
55 mg/hr	55 mL/hr
60 mg/hr	60 mL/hr
65 mg/hr	65 mL/hr
70 mg/hr	70 mL/hr
75 mg/hr	75 mL/hr

Aminophylline (Theophylline)

Amiodarone (Cordarone)

USES

1. Initiation of treatment and prophylaxis of recurring ventricular fibrillation and unstable ventricular tachycardia in patients refractory to other therapy.
2. In patients for whom oral amiodarone is indicated but who are NPO.

SOLUTION PREPARATION

Loading dose: Amiodarone is added to D5W bag (150 mg in 100 mL). *Maintenance dose:* 900 mg amiodarone is added to 500 mL D5W in a glass bottle.

DOSE

1. Infuse 150 mg over 10 minutes (15 mg/min). Prepare solution with 150 mg amiodarone in 100-mL D5W bag. The initial infusion rate is not >30 mg/min.
2. Follow with a slow infusion of 360 mg over the next 6 hours (1 mg/min). Prepare solution with 900 mg amiodarone in 500 mL D5W glass bottle.
3. Follow with a maintenance infusion of 540 mg over the remaining 18 hours (0.5 mg/min).
4. After the first 24 hours: 0.5 mg/min continuous infusion. If IV concentration is >2 mg/mL, it should be administered through a central venous catheter with in-line filter. (For >2 mg/mL, administer via central venous catheter only.)
5. If breakthrough episodes of ventricular fibrillation or tachycardia should occur, an additional infusion of 150 mg over 10 minutes may be administered (150 mg in 100 mL D5W).
6. When switching from IV to PO, use the following as a guide:
   a. <1week IV → 800-1600 mg/day
   b. 1-3 weeks IV → 600-800 mg/day
   c. >3 weeks IV → 400 mg/day
7. During cardiac arrest, 300 mg (2 ampules 150 mg each) may be given IV push. May repeat 150-mg IV push in 3-5 minutes, up to a maximum cumulative dose of 2.2 g IV in 24 hours.

WARNINGS

1. Although IV amiodarone has been used safely in some patients with acute myocardial infarction (AMI), it is clearly a negative inotrope. Use cautiously in patients with left ventricular dysfunction.
2. Hypotension is the main complication of IV therapy; therefore use with caution in hypotensive patients.
3. Marked cardiomegaly, particularly resulting from myocardiopathy, is a relative contraindication to IV use of amiodarone.
4. Use cautiously in patients with thyroid dysfunction. Amiodarone has been reported to produce hypothyroidism or hyperthyroidism.
5. Because of extensive tissue distribution and prolonged elimination period, the time at which a life-threatening arrhythmia will recur following discontinued therapy or an interaction with subsequent treatment may be unpredictable. Patients must be observed carefully when other antiarrhythmic agents are substituted after amiodarone is stopped.

ADVERSE REACTIONS

The incidence of side effects increases over time; many adverse drug reactions (ADRs) may be related to the total dose administered over time (i.e., accumulation).

1. *Cardiovascular:* Sinus bradycardia, hypotension, heart block, proarrhythmic effects.
2. *Pulmonary:* Within the first few weeks, may present with acute onset of nonspecific symptoms (e.g., fever, shortness of breath, and cough). These are probably symptoms of a hypersensitivity reaction associated with an eosinophilic lung infiltrate (e.g., pulmonary fibrosis, interstitial pneumonitis).
3. *Thyroid:* Interferes with $T_4 \rightarrow T_3$ conversion (hypothyroidism occurs more often than hyperthyroidism).
4. *GI:* Nausea/vomiting, anorexia, abdominal pain, and constipation.
5. *Hepatic:* Abnormal liver function tests, especially elevated aminotransferase and alkaline phosphatase levels, $\approx 25\%$ of patients. Increased prothrombin time (PT)/international normalized ratio (INR).

Amiodarone (Cordarone)

Amiodarone (Cordarone)

6. *Dermatologic:* Allergic rash, photosensitivity, and unusual blue-gray skin discoloration.
7. *Neurologic:* Tremor, ataxia, peripheral neuropathy, fatigue, and weakness.
8. *Ophthalmologic:* High occurrence of corneal microdeposits caused by the secretion of amiodarone by the lacrimal gland with accumulation on corneal surface. This does not seem to affect vision and is reversible once the drug is discontinued.
9. *Hematologic:* Thrombocytopenia $\approx$ <1%.

INCOMPATIBILITY

Aminophylline	Heparin
Cefazolin	Sodium bicarbonate

COMPATIBILITY

Amikacin	Metaraminol
Bretylium	Metronidazole
Clindamycin	Midazolam
Dobutamine	Morphine
Dopamine	Nitroglycerin
Doxycycline	Norepinephrine
Erythromycin	Penicillin G
Esmolol	Phentolamine
Gentamicin	Phenylephrine
Insulin	Potassium chloride
Isoproterenol	Procainamide
Labetalol	Tobramycin
Lidocaine	Vancomycin

Drug Interactions

Drug	Interaction effect
Warfarin	Increased anticoagulation effect
Beta-blockers	Beta-blocker effects are enhanced
Calcium channel blockers	Additive effects of both drugs are enhanced, resulting in reduced cardiac sinus and AV nodal conduction, and contractility
Digoxin	Increased digoxin concentrations, thus increasing toxic potential
Flecainide	Increased flecainide concentrations
Phenytoin	Increased phenytoin concentrations
Procainamide	Increased procainamide concentrations
Quinidine	Increased quinidine concentrations, which can cause fatal cardiac arrhythmias

Amiodarone (Cordarone)

Amiodarone (Cordarone)

NURSING CONSIDERATIONS

1. Consult the Amiodarone Drip Rate Calculation Chart to determine the drip rate.
2. Muscle weakness may present a great hazard for ambulation.
3. Give PO dosage with food.
4. Monitor ECG and rhythm throughout therapy.
5. Assess patient for signs of lethargy, edema of the hands and feet, weight loss, and pulmonary toxicity (e.g., shortness of breath, cough, rales, fever, pulmonary function tests).

Amiodarone Drip Rate Calculation Chart

Dose	Concentration	Infusion rate
15 mg/min	150 mg amiodarone /100 mL D5W = 1.5 mg/1 mL D5W	600 mL/hr
1 mg/min	900 mg/500 mL D5W = 1.8 mg/1 mL D5W	33 mL/hr × 6 hr
0.5 mg/min	900 mg/500 mL D5W = 1.8 mg/1 mL D5W	17 mL/hr × 18 hr
After the First 24 hr		
0.5 mg/min	600 mg/500 mL = 1.2 mg/mL	25 mL/hr

Amiodarone (Cordarone)

Argatroban (Acova)

USES

1. Anticoagulation for prophylaxis or treatment of thrombosis in patients with heparin-induced thrombocytopenia (HIT).
2. Anticoagulant therapy in patients who have or are at risk for HIT undergoing percutaneous coronary intervention (PCI).

SOLUTION PREPARATION

Argatroban is available in 250-mg (2.5-mL) single use vials and should be added to 250-mL NS, D5W, or LR, to a final concentration of 1 mg/mL. Alternatively, 500 mg (5 mL) may be added to 500 mL of diluent. The final solution must be mixed by repeated inversion of the diluent bag for 1 minute. Upon preparation, the solution may show slight but brief haziness because of the formation of microprecipitates that rapidly dissolve upon mixing.

DOSES

The recommended initial dose of argatroban for adult patients without hepatic impairment is 2 mcg/kg/min, administered as a continuous intravenous infusion.
Dosage adjustment: After the initial dose, the dose of argatroban can be adjusted as clinically indicated (not to exceed 10 mcg/kg/min), until the steady-state aPTT is 1.5 to 3 times the initial baseline value, usually about 55-80 seconds (not to exceed 100 seconds).

WARNINGS

1. Heparin must be discontinued before administration of argatroban.
2. A baseline aPTT should be obtained before initiating therapy.
3. Patients with hepatic impairment require a dosage adjustment.
4. Doses >10 mcg/kg/min should not be administered.
5. Contraindicated in overt bleeding.
6. Hemorrhage can occur at any site in the body; an unexplained fall in hematocrit or blood pressure should be evaluated for bleeding.
7. Use extreme caution in the following instances: Severe hypertension; immediately following

lumbar puncture; spinal anesthesia; major surgery, especially involving the brain, spinal cord or eye; hematologic conditions associated with increased bleeding tendencies such as congenital or acquired bleeding disorders and GI lesions such as ulcerations.

ADVERSE REACTIONS
1. Bleeding (5.3%) is the most common serious reaction.
2. Hypotension (7.2%), fever (6.9%), diarrhea (6.2%), nausea (4.8%), and vomiting (4.2%) have been reported.

INCOMPATIBILITIES
No compatibility studies have been done with argatroban. Argatroban should be infused in alone and not mixed with other agents.

NURSING CONSIDERATIONS
1. Monitor therapy using the aPTT. The aPTT typically reaches steady-state effect levels within 1 to 3 hours after initiation.
2. Dose adjustment may be required to attain the target aPTT. Check the aPTT 2 hours after initiation of therapy or dosage adjustment to confirm that the patient has attained the desired therapeutic range (1.5 to 3 times control, usually about 55-80 seconds).
3. For conversion to oral therapy with warfarin, maintain argatroban infusion until INR is greater than 4. Combination therapy with argatroban and warfarin does produce a combined effect on laboratory measurement of INR. Once INR is greater than 4, then stop the infusion, repeat INR 4-6 hours later; if INR is between 2 and 3, maintain warfarin monotherapy.

Argatroban (Acova)

Argatroban Dosing Charts
Usual Dose 2 mcg/kg/min
Mix 250 mg in 250 mL NS
Final Concentration: 1 mg/mL

Body weight	Initial infusion rate	Initial infusion rate for hepatic impairment (0.5 mcg/kg/min)	Maximum dose 10 mcg/kg/min Maximum infusion rate
50 kg	6 mL/hr	1.5 mL/hr	30 mL/hr
60 kg	7 mL/hr	1.8 mL/hr	35 mL/hr
70 kg	8 mL/hr	2 mL/hr	40 mL/hr
80 kg	10 mL/hr	2.5 mL/hr	50 mL/hr
90 kg	11 mL/hr	2.8 mL/hr	55 mL/hr
100 kg	12 mL/hr	3 mL/hr	60 mL/hr
110 kg	13 mL/hr	3.3 mL/hr	65 mL/hr
120 kg	14 mL/hr	3.5 mL/hr	70 mL/hr
130 kg	16 mL/hr	4 mL/hr	80 mL/hr
140 kg	17 mL/hr	4.3 mL/hr	85 mL/hr

Argatroban Dosing Adjustments

HIT patients	HIT patients with *renal* impairment	HIT patients with *hepatic* impairment
Initiate at 2 mcg/kg/min	No dosage adjustment required	Initiate at 0.5 mcg/kg/min
Titrate until steady-state aPTT is 1.5 to 3 times baseline value		Titrate until steady-state aPTT is 1.5 to 3 times baseline value

Argatroban (Acova)

Atracurium (Tracrium)

USES

Skeletal muscle relaxation during mechanical ventilation to prevent ventilator resistance and/or decreased energy expenditure states. Paralysis of skeletal muscles requires that patients be intubated and on mechanical ventilation.

SOLUTION PREPARATION

To prepare Tracrium infusion, add 250 mg (25 mL) Tracrium to 250 mL D5W. Final concentration: 1 mg/mL.

DOSE

Continuous infusion
1. Start 0.5 mg/kg/hr (rate rounded off to nearest 5 mg/hr).
2. If ineffective, give 10-mg bolus undiluted and increase rate of infusion by 5 mg/hr.
3. Increase dose as needed to achieve desired degree of neuromuscular blockade.

WARNINGS

1. Sedation should be ordered and given in addition to atracurium because it does not alter the level of consciousness and does not relieve pain.
2. Tracrium drip may be interrupted to assess neurologic status based on physician's orders. Neurologic assessment will include responsiveness, orientation, extremity movement, and pupillary reaction.
3. If drip is interrupted, patient should be given 10-mg bolus and resume prior rate (mg/hr).

ADVERSE REACTIONS

1. Hypotension, laryngospasm, rash and urticaria, bradycardia, tachycardia
2. Flushing (1%-10%)

INCOMPATIBILITY

Aminophylline   Propofol
Diazepam   Thiopental

COMPATIBILITY

Bretylium
Cefazolin
Cefuroxime
Cimetidine
Dobutamine
Dopamine
Epinephrine
Esmolol
Etomidate
Fentanyl
Gentamicin
Heparin
Hydrocortisone
Isoproterenol
Lidocaine
Lorazepam
Midazolam
Milrinone
Morphine
Nitroglycerin
Procainamide
Ranitidine
Sodium nitroprusside
Trimethoprim/sulfa
Vancomycin

NURSING CONSIDERATIONS

1. Use infusion control device and monitor ECG, respirations, and vital signs continuously.
2. Monitor for malignant hyperthermia.
3. Tachyphylaxis is possible in long-term use.
4. Anticholinesterase reversal agents, endotracheal intubation equipment, and mechanical ventilation equipment should be available.
5. No dosage reductions are needed for renal or hepatic insufficiency.
6. The desired level of neuromuscular blockade is usually measured by train of four peripheral neurostimulator assessment. Typically, the goal of therapy is 0/4 train of four (100% blocked) to 2/4 train of four (75% blocked). Usually, this is assessed every 15 minutes during titration and at least every 4 hours during maintenance infusion.
7. A "sedation holiday" or temporary removal of the infusion may be necessary for all patients on therapy for more than 48 hours to assess the patient for continued need and to conduct a neurologic exam.

Atracurium (Tracrium)

Atracurium (Tracrium)

Atracurium (Tracrium) Drip Rate Calculation Chart
Tracrium 250 mg Added to 250 mL (Concentration: 1 mg/mL or 1000 mcg/mL)

Patient weight	Dose (0.5 mg/kg/hr)	Infusion rate
50 kg	25 mg/hr	25 mL/hr
60 kg	30 mg/hr	30 mL/hr
70 kg	35 mg/hr	35 mL/hr
80 kg	40 mg/hr	40 mL/hr
90 kg	45 mg/hr	45 mL/hr

Bivalirudin (Angiomax)

USES

For the replacement of heparin in patients undergoing percutaneous coronary intervention (PCI) who are at a high risk for bleeding or thrombotic complications. Angiomax is a bivalent, direct thrombin inhibitor that provides rapid and reversible anticoagulant activity during PCI.

SOLUTION PREPARATION

1. Reconstitute 250-mg vial with 5 mL of sterile water for injection and dissolve powder by gently swirling vial (do not shake).
2. Withdraw entire contents of the vial and add to a 50-ml bag of desired IV fluid. Resulting concentration of solution is 5 mg/mL. *Compatible solutions:* D5W, NS.
3. Use within 24 hours. May be stored at room temperature.

DOSE

Initial bolus dose of 1 mg/kg followed by an infusion of 2.5 mg/kg/hr for an initial 4-hour period (see dosing chart). Discontinue after PCI unless there are complications that require prolonged anticoagulation. May be continued at 2.5 mg/kg/hr for the completion of the bag ($\approx$4 hr). After 4 hours, the dose of 0.2 mg/kg/hr may be continued up to 20 hours if needed.

Dosage Adjustment

Infusion rate should be decreased as follows in patients with moderate to severe renal impairment.

Maintenance dose	Creatinine clearance
1.4 mg/kg/hr	30-59 mL/min
0.7 mg/kg/hr	10-29 mL/min
0.2 mg/kg/hr	<10 mL/min

Bivalirudin (Angiomax)

Bivalirudin (Angiomax)

WARNINGS
Should not be used in patients with active bleeding disorders or known sensitivity to Angiomax.

ADVERSE REACTIONS
The main adverse reaction to Angiomax is bleeding, but this has been shown to be less than with heparin.

INCOMPATIBILITY (INCLUDING Y-SITE)
Alteplase (tPA)
Amiodarone hydrochloride
Amphotericin B
Chlorpromazine hydrochloride
Diazepam
Prochlorperazine
Reteplase (rtPA)
Streptokinase
Vancomycin hydrochloride

COMPATIBILITY
Dexamethasone
Digoxin
Diphenhydramine
Dobutamine
Dopamine
Epinephrine
Eptifibatide
Esmolol
Furosemide
Heparin
Hydrocortisone
Lidocaine
Meperidine
Methylprednisolone
Midazolam
Morphine
Nitroglycerin
Potassium chloride
Sodium bicarbonate
Tirofiban
Verapamil

NURSING CONSIDERATIONS
1. Sheath removal may be performed using a time-based procedure instead of serial ACT monitoring. Angiomax achieves rapid hemostasis at the groin site with 10-15 minutes of manual pressure and may obviate the need for closure devices.

Renal function	Time to sheath removal	Estimated Angiomax serum levels
CrCl ≥ 30 mL/min	1 hour	<2 mcg/mL
CrCl 10-30 mL/min	2-2.5 hours	<2 mcg/mL

2. Patients previously treated with unfractionated heparin prior to arrival in the cath lab can be switched to bivalirudin after heparin has been discontinued for approximately 30 minutes.

3. Low molecular weight heparin (LMWH) should be discontinued for *at least 8 hours* prior to bivalirudin administration.

Bivalirudin (Angiomax)

Bivalirudin (Angiomax) Dosing Chart
250 mg in 50 mL NS or D5W
Final Concentration: 5 mg/mL

Patient weight	IV Bolus dose (1 mg/kg)	Infusion rate (2.5 mg/kg/hr)	Low-rate infusion (0.2 mg/kg/hr)
58-62 kg	12 mL	30 mL/hr	2.4 mL/hr
63-67 kg	13 mL	32.5 mL/hr	2.6 mL/hr
68-72 kg	14 mL	35 mL/hr	2.8 mL/hr
73-77 kg	15 mL	37.5 mL/hr	3 mL/hr
78-82 kg	16 mL	40 mL/hr	3.2 mL/hr
83-87 kg	17 mL	42.5 mL/hr	3.4 mL/hr
88-92 kg	18 mL	45 mL/hr	3.6 mL/hr
93-97 kg	19 mL	47.5 mL/hr	3.8 mL/hr
98-102 kg	20 mL	50 mL/hr	4 mL/hr
103-107 kg	21 mL	52.5 mL/hr	4.2 mL/hr
108-112 kg	22 mL	55 mL/hr	4.4 mL/hr
113-117 kg	23 mL	57.5 mL/hr	4.6 mL/hr
118-122 kg	24 mL	60 mL/hr	4.8 mL/hr
123-127 kg	25 mL	62.5 mL/hr	5 mL/hr
128-132 kg	26 mL	65 mL/hr	5.2 mL/hr

Cisatracurium (Nimbex)

USES
Skeletal muscle relaxation during mechanical ventilation to prevent ventilator resistance and/or decreased energy expenditure states. Paralysis of skeletal muscles requires that patients must be intubated and on mechanical ventilation.

SOLUTION PREPARATION
To prepare Nimbex infusion, add 250 mg (25 × 5 mL each vial) Nimbex to 125 mL D5W (waste 125 mL D5W from a 250-mL bag). Final concentration: 1 mg/mL.

DOSE
Continuous infusion
1. Start 3.0 mcg/kg/min (range 0.5-10 mcg/kg/min).
2. Titrate dose to effect.
3. Increase dose as needed to achieve desired degree of neuromuscular blockade.

WARNINGS
1. Sedation should be ordered and given in addition to the cisatracurium because it does not alter the level of consciousness and does not relieve pain.
2. Nimbex drip may be interrupted to assess neurologic status based on physician's orders. Neurologic assessment will include responsiveness, orientation, extremity movement, and pupillary reaction.

ADVERSE REACTIONS
Bradycardia (0.4%), hypotension (0.2%), flushing (0.2%), bronchospasm (0.2%), rash (0.1%)

INCOMPATIBILITY
Acyclovir
Aminophylline
Amphotericin B
Ampicillin

Ampicillin/sulbactam
Cefazolin
Cefotaxime
Cefotetan

Cefoxitin
Ceftazidime
Cefuroxime
Diazepam
Diprivan
Furosemide
Ganciclovir
Heparin

Ketorolac
Methylprednisolone
Nitroprusside
Piperacillin
Thiopental
Ticarcillin/clavulanate
Trimethoprim/sulfa
Zosyn

COMPATIBILITY (VIA Y-SITE ADMINISTRATION)

Alfentanil
Amikacin
Aztreonam
Bretylium
Bumetanide
Buprenorphine
Butorphanol
Calcium gluconate
Ceftriaxone
Chlorpromazine
Cimetidine

Ciprofloxacin
Clindamycin
Dexamethasone
Digoxin
Diphenhydramine
Dobutamine
Dopamine
Doxycycline
Droperidol
Enalaprilat
Epinephrine

Esmolol
Famotidine
Fentanyl
Fluconazole
Gatifloxacin
Gentamicin
Haloperidol
Hydrocortisone
Hydromorphone
Hydroxyzine
Imipenem/cilastatin
Inamrinone
Isoproterenol
Ketorolac
Lidocaine
Linezolid
Lorazepam
Magnesium sulfate
Mannitol
Meperidine
Metoclopramide
Metronidazole

Midazolam
Minocycline
Morphine
Nalbuphine
Nitroglycerin
Norepinephrine
Ofloxacin
Ondansetron
Phenylephrine
Potassium chloride
Procainamide
Prochlorperazine
Promethazine
Ranitidine
Remifentanil
Sufentanil
Theophylline
Ticarcillin
Tobramycin
Vancomycin
Zidovudine

Cisatracurium (Nimbex)

Cisatracurium (Nimbex)

NURSING CONSIDERATIONS

1. Use infusion control device and monitor ECG, respirations, and vital signs continuously.
2. Monitor for malignant hyperthermia.
3. Tachyphylaxis is possible in long-term use.
4. Anticholinesterase reversal agents, endotracheal intubation equipment, and mechanical ventilation equipment should be available.
5. No dosage reductions are needed for renal or hepatic insufficiency.
6. The desired level of neuromuscular blockade is usually measured by train of four peripheral neurostimulator assessment. Typically, the goal of therapy is 0/4 train of four (100% blocked) to 2/4 train of four (75% blocked). Usually, this is assessed every 15 minutes during titration and at least every 4 hours during maintenance infusion.
7. A "sedation holiday" or temporary removal of the infusion may be necessary for all patients on therapy for greater than 48 hours to assess the patient for continued need and to conduct a neurologic exam.

Cisatracurium (Nimbex) Drip Rate Calculation Chart
Nimbex 250 mg in 250 mL (Concentration: 1 mg/mL or 1000 mcg/mL)

Patient weight	Dose (3.0 mcg/kg/min)	Infusion rate
50 kg	9 mg/hr	9 mL/hr
60 kg	11 mg/hr	11 mL/hr
70 kg	13 mg/hr	13 mL/hr
80 kg	14 mg/hr	14 mL/hr
90 kg	16 mg/hr	16 mL/hr

Cisatracurium (Nimbex)

Dexmedetomidine (Precedex)

USES
Indicated for short-term use as a sedative for patients undergoing mechanical ventilation in the ICU and cardiac surgery unit (CSU) setting.

SOLUTION PREPARATION
Dilute 2 mL dexmedetomidine into 48 mL NS before IV administration for any purpose.

DOSE
The usual starting dose is 0.3-0.4 mcg/kg/hr, followed by a maintenance infusion of 0.2-0.7 mcg/kg/hr. The rate of maintenance should be adjusted to achieve the desired level of sedation.

Precedex should be used with midazolam or morphine and never used alone.

WARNINGS
1. Patients should be continuously monitored while receiving dexmedetomidine because of clinically significant episodes of bradycardia and sinus arrest.
2. Caution should be exercised when administering dexmedetomidine to patients with advanced heart block.
3. Transient hypertension has been observed primarily during the loading dose in association with the initial peripheral vasoconstrictive effects of dexmedetomidine.
4. Abrupt discontinuation can result in nervousness, agitation, and headaches accompanied by a rapid rise in BP and elevated catecholamine concentrations in the plasma.

ADVERSE REACTIONS
1. *Incidence >10%:* Hypotension, hypertension, nausea
2. *Incidence 1%-10%:* Bradycardia, atrial fibrillation, hypoxia, anemia, pain, pleural effusion, infection, leukocytosis, oliguria, pulmonary edema, thirst
3. *Incidence <1%:* Fever, hyperpyrexia, hypovolemia, light anesthesia, pain, rigors, BP fluctuation, heart disorder, aggravated hypertension, dizziness,

headache, neuralgia, neuritis, speech disorder, abdominal pain, diarrhea, vomiting, arrhythmias, atrioventricular (AV) block, cardiac arrest, extrasystoles, atrial fibrillation, heart block, T-wave inversion, tachycardia, supraventricular tachycardia, increased GGT, increased SGOT, increased SGPT, acidosis, respiratory acidosis, hyperkalemia, increased alkaline phosphatase, agitation, confusion, delirium, hallucination, illusion, somnolence, anemia, apnea, bronchospasm, dyspnea, hypercapnia, hypoventilation, hypoxia, pulmonary congestion, increased sweating, photopsia, abnormal vision

INCOMPATIBILITY

Blood: Serum or plasma

COMPATIBILITY

Atracurium besylate
Atropine sulfate
Fentanyl citrate
Glycopyrrolate bromide
20% Mannitol

Midazolam
Mivacurium chloride
Morphine sulfate
Normal saline

NURSING CONSIDERATIONS

1. Use administration components made with synthetic or coated natural rubber gaskets.
2. Products should be inspected visually for particulate matter and discoloration before administration.
3. Consult the Dexmedetomidine Drip Rate Calculation Chart to determine the drip rate.
4. Safety and effectiveness of dexmedetomidine has not been evaluated in infusions over 24 hours; however, it has been used for up to 9 days in some patients.

Dexmedetomidine (Precedex)

Dexmedetomidine (Precedex) Drip Rate Calculation Chart
Precedex 50 mL Minibag (Concentration: 4 mcg/mL)

Patient weight	Common infusion rates					
	0.2 mg/kg/hr	0.3 mg/kg/hr	0.4 mg/kg/hr	0.5 mg/kg/hr	0.6 mg/kg/hr	0.7 mg/kg/hr
50 kg	2 mL/hr	4 mL/hr	5 mL/hr	6 mL/hr	8 mL/hr	9 mL/hr
60 kg	3 mL/hr	5 mL/hr	6 mL/hr	8 mL/hr	9 mL/hr	11 mL/hr
70 kg	4 mL/hr	5 mL/hr	7 mL/hr	9 mL/hr	11 mL/hr	12 mL/hr
80 kg	4 mL/hr	6 mL/hr	8 mL/hr	10 mL/hr	12 mL/hr	14 mL/hr
90 kg	5 mL/hr	7 mL/hr	9 mL/hr	11 mL/hr	14 mL/hr	16 mL/hr
100 kg	5 mL/hr	8 mL/hr	10 mL/hr	13 mL/hr	15 mL/hr	18 mL/hr

Dose (mcg/kg/min) = CF × Rate (mL/hr). Usual dose: 0.2-0.7 mcg/kg/hr. Starting dose: 0.3-0.4 mcg/kg/hr.

Calculation Factors (CF) by Patient Weight (50-100 kg)

kg	50	55	60	65	70	75	80	85	90	95	100
CF	0.10		0.07		0.05		0.05		0.04		0.04

Diltiazem (Cardizem)

USES
1. Paroxysmal supraventricular tachycardia.
2. Atrial flutter or fibrillation; temporary control of rapid ventricular rate.

SOLUTION PREPARATION
To prepare diltiazem infusion, add 125 mg (5 × 25-mg vials) diltiazem to 100 mL D5W. **Final concentration:** 1 mg/mL.

DOSE
1. Bolus dose
   a. Initial dose of 0.25 mg/kg (average: 20 mg) given over 2 minutes.
   b. If inadequate results after 15 minutes, additional bolus of 0.35 mg/kg (average: 25 mg) may be given.
2. Continuous infusion
   a. Give bolus as described above, immediately followed by a continuous infusion of 5-10 mg/hr.
   b. Infusion may be increased to 15 mg/hr if further reduction in HR is required.
   c. Infusions longer than 24 hours or >15 mg/hr are not recommended.

WARNINGS
1. Diltiazem may prolong atrioventricular (AV) node conduction and rarely may cause second- or third-degree heart block. It is contraindicated in patients with sick sinus syndrome or heart block unless functioning ventricular pacemaker is present.
2. Monitor response and possibly decrease dose in patients with liver failure. Rare instances of acute hepatic injury have occurred with diltiazem injection.
3. May cause hypotension; use with caution in hemodynamically compromised patients and those taking drugs that decrease peripheral resistance, intravascular volume, myocardial contractility, or conduction.

ADVERSE REACTIONS

1. *Cardiovascular:* Hypotension—treat with saline or Trendelenburg position if required. Vasodilation (flushing) may occur. Atrial flutter, atrioventricular (AV) block, bradycardia, chest pain, congestive heart failure (CHF), and ventricular arrhythmias have been reported.
2. *GI:* Constipation, nausea, vomiting, elevated liver function tests.
3. *CNS:* Dizziness, paresthesia, headache.
4. *Other:* Amblyopia, dry mouth, dyspnea, edema.

INCOMPATIBILITY

Acetazolamide
Acyclovir
Aminophylline
Ampicillin
Diazepam
Hydrocortisone
Insulin
Lasix
Methylprednisolone
Phenytoin
Procainamide
Rifampin
Sodium bicarbonate
Thiopental

COMPATIBILITY

Aminophylline
Albumin
Amikacin
Amphotericin B
Aztreonam
Bretylium
Bumetanide
Cefazolin
Cefotaxime
Cefoxitin
Ceftazidime
Ceftriaxone
Cefuroxime
Cimetidine
Ciprofloxacin
Clindamycin
Digoxin
Dobutamine
Dopamine
Doxycycline
Epinephrine
Erythromycin
Esmolol
Fentanyl
Fluconazole
Gentamicin
Heparin
Hetastarch
Hydromorphone
Imipenem/cilastatin
Insulin
Labetalol
Lidocaine
Lorazepam
Meperidine
Metoclopramide
Metronidazole
Midazolam

Diltiazem (Cardizem)

Diltiazem (Cardizem)

Milrinone
Morphine
Multivitamins
Nicardipine
Oxacillin
Penicillin G
Pentamidine
Piperacillin
Potassium chloride
Potassium phosphate

Ranitidine
Nitroglycerin
Nitroprusside
Norepinephrine
Theophylline
Ticarcillin/clavulanate
Tobramycin
Trimethoprim/sulfa
Vancomycin
Vecuronium

NURSING CONSIDERATIONS

1. Consult the Diltiazem Drip Rate Calculation Chart to determine the drip rate.
2. Diltiazem should be administered by an IV pump to ensure controlled infusion.
3. Closely monitor and document changes in BP, HR, or in the rhythm strip. Document BP at least every hour.

Diltiazem (Cardizem) Drip Rate Calculation Chart
Diltiazem 125 mg Added to 100 mL (Concentration: 1 mg/mL)

Dose	Infusion rate
5 mg/hr	5 mL/hr
6 mg/hr	6 mL/hr
7 mg/hr	7 mL/hr
8 mg/hr	8 mL/hr
9 mg/hr	9 mL/hr
10 mg/hr	10 mL/hr
11 mg/hr	11 mL/hr
12 mg/hr	12 mL/hr
13 mg/hr	13 mL/hr
14 mg/hr	14 mL/hr
15 mg/hr	15 mL/hr

Diltiazem (Cardizem)

Dobutamine (Dobutrex)

USES

1. To increase cardiac output in the short-term treatment of patients with cardiac decompensation resulting from depressed contractility (inotropic support).
2. Cardiogenic shock.

SOLUTION PREPARATION

Premixed dobutamine 500 mg/250 mL in D5W.
Final concentration: 2 mg/mL.

DOSE

Usual dose is 2.5-10 mcg/kg/min; rarely up to 40 mcg/kg/min may be given. Infusion is titrated until optimal response is obtained (dose increased 2 mcg/kg/min at 15- to 20-minute intervals). Onset of action is usually within 2 minutes, and peak effects usually occur within 10 minutes of initiation.

WARNINGS

1. Hypovolemia should be corrected before use.
2. In the presence of atrial fibrillation, digoxin is usually given before dobutamine initiation to prevent development of a rapid ventricular response.
3. Dobutamine is contraindicated in patients with idiopathic hypertropic subaortic stenosis (IHSS).
4. Dobutamine should be used with extreme caution after myocardial infarction (MI) or in patients with marked mechanical obstruction (e.g., severe valvular aortic stenosis).
5. Use with caution in patients receiving halothane or cyclopropane anesthesia.
6. Dobutamine effects are antagonized by beta-blockers.

ADVERSE REACTIONS

1. Increased HR, increased BP, and ectopic beats. These are usually dose related and may respond to a dosage decrease or a temporary discontinuation of the drug.
2. Increase in AV conduction.
3. Angina, nausea, vomiting, tingling, paresthesia, dyspnea, headache, mild leg cramps.

INCOMPATIBILITY

Acyclovir
Alteplase
Aminophylline
Amphotericin B
Calcium
Cefazolin
Cefepime
Diazepam
Digoxin
Foscarnet
Furosemide
Heparin
Hydrocortisone
Indomethacin
Insulin
Magnesium sulfate
Midazolam
Phenytoin
Piperacillin/tazobactam
Sodium bicarbonate
Thiopental

COMPATIBILITY

Amiodarone
Atracurium
Aztreonam
Bretylium
Cladribine
Calcium chloride
Calcium gluconate
Ciprofloxacin
Cisatracurium
Diazepam
Diltiazem
Docetaxel
Dopamine
Doxorubicin
Enalaprilat
Epinephrine
Etoposide
Famotidine
Fentanyl
Fluconazole
Gatifloxacin
Gemcitabine
Granisetron
Haloperidol
Hydromorphone
Inamrinone
Insulin
Isoproterenol
Labetalol
Levofloxacin
Lidocaine
Linezolid
Lorazepam
Magnesium sulfate
Meperidine
Milrinone
Morphine
Nicardipine
Nitroglycerin
Nitroprusside

Dobutamine (Dobutrex)

Norepinephrine
Pancuronium
Potassium chloride
Procainamide
Propofol
Ranitidine
Remifentanil
Streptokinase

Tacrolimus
Theophylline
Thiotepa
Tolazoline
Vecuronium
Verapamil
Zidovudine

NURSING CONSIDERATIONS

1. The drip may turn a light pink several hours after mixing, but stability or potency is not altered.
2. An accurate weight should be obtained before administration of dobutamine.
3. Consult the Dobutamine Drip Rate Calculation Chart to determine the drip rate.
4. Except in cardiac arrest situations, dobutamine should be administered via an IV pump to ensure controlled infusion.
5. Closely monitor and document changes in BP, HR, or the rhythm strip. Document BP at least every hour. Pulmonary wedge pressure and cardiac output monitoring is desirable.

Dobutamine (Dobutrex) Drip Rate Calculation Chart—
Patient Weight 35-80 kg (77-176 lbs)
Concentration: 2 mg/mL (500 mg/250 mL)

lbs	77	88	99	110	121	132	143	154	165	176
kg	35	40	45	50	55	60	65	70	75	80
mL/hr										
5	4.8	4.2	3.7	3.3	3	2.8	2.6	2.4	2.2	2.1
10	9.5	8.3	7.4	6.7	6.1	5.6	5.1	4.8	4.4	4.2
15	14.3	12.5	11.1	10	9.1	8.3	7.7	7.1	6.7	6.3
20	19	16.7	14.8	13.3	12.2	11.1	10.3	9.5	8.9	8.3
25	23.8	20.8	18.5	16.7	15.2	13.9	12.8	11.9	11.1	10.4
30	28.6	25	22.2	20	18.2	16.7	15.7	14.3	13.3	12.5
35	33.3	29.2	25.9	23.3	21.2	19.4	17.9	16.7	15.6	14.6
40	38.1	33.3	29.6	26.7	24.2	22.2	20.8	19	17.8	16.7
45	42.9	37.5	33.3	30	27.5	25	23.1	21.4	20	18.6
50	47.6	41.7	37	33.3	30.3	27.8	25.6	23.8	22.2	20.8
55	52.4	45.8	40.7	36.7	33.3	30.6	28.2	26.2	24.4	22.9
60	57.1	50	44.4	40	36.4	33.3	30.8	28.6	26.7	25
65	61.9	54.2	48.1	43.3	39.4	36.1	33.3	31	28.9	27.1

Continued

Dobutamine (Dobutrex)

Dobutamine (Dobutrex)

Dobutamine (Dobutrex) Drip Rate Calculation Chart—Patient Weight 35-80 kg (77-176 lbs)—cont'd
Concentration: 2 mg/mL (500 mg/250 mL)

lbs	77	88	99	110	121	132	143	154	165	176
kg	35	40	45	50	55	60	65	70	75	80
mL/hr										
70	66.7	58.3	51.9	46.7	42.4	38.8	35.9	33.3	31.1	29.2
75	71.4	62.5	55.6	50	45.5	41.7	38.5	35.7	33.3	31.3
80	76.2	66.7	59.3	53.3	48.5	44.4	41	38.1	35.6	33.3
85	81	70.8	63	56.7	51.5	47.2	43.6	40.5	37.8	35.4
90	85.7	75	66.7	60	54.5	50	46.2	43	40	37.5

Dose (mcg/kg/min) = CF × Rate (mL/hr).

Calculation Factors (CF) by Patient Weight (35-80 kg)

kg	35	40	45	50	55	60	65	70	75	80
CF	0.952	0.833	0.741	0.667	0.606	0.556	0.513	0.476	0.444	0.417

Dobutamine (Dobutrex) Drip Rate Calculation Chart—
Patient Weight 85-140 kg (199-297 lbs)
Concentration: 2 mg/mL (500 mg/250 mL)

| lbs | 189 | 199 | 209 | 220 | 231 | 242 | 253 | 264 | 275 | 286 | 297 |
kg	85	90	95	100	105	110	115	120	125	130	140
mL/hr											
5	2	1.8	1.8	1.7	1.6	1.5	1.5	1.4	1.4	1.3	1.2
10	3.9	3.7	3.5	3.3	3.2	3	2.9	2.8	2.7	2.5	2.4
15	5.9	5.6	5.3	5	4.8	4.5	4.3	4.2	4	3.8	3.6
20	7.8	7.4	7	6.7	6.3	6.1	5.8	5.5	5.4	5.1	4.8
25	9.8	9.3	8.8	8.3	7.9	7.6	7.2	6.9	6.6	6.4	5.9
30	11.8	11.1	10.5	10	9.5	9.1	8.6	8.3	8	7.7	7.1
35	13.7	13	12.3	11.7	11.1	10.6	10.1	9.7	9.4	9	8.3
40	15.7	14.8	14	13.3	12.7	12.1	11.6	11.1	10.7	10.2	9.5
45	17.6	16.7	15.8	15	14.3	13.6	13	12.5	11.9	11.5	10.7
50	19.6	18.5	17.5	16.7	15.9	15.2	14.5	13.9	13.3	12.8	11.8
55	21.6	20.4	19.3	18.3	17.5	16.7	15.9	15.3	14.6	14.1	13.1
60	23.5	22.2	21.1	20	19	18.2	17.4	16.7	16	15.4	14.3
65	25.5	24.1	22.8	21.7	20.6	19.7	18.9	18	17.4	16.7	15.5

Dobutamine (Dobutrex)

Dobutamine (Dobutrex)

Dobutamine (Dobutrex) Drip Rate Calculation Chart—
Patient Weight 85-140 kg (199-297 lbs)—cont'd
Concentration: 2 mg/mL (500 mg/250 mL)

lbs	189	199	209	220	231	242	253	264	275	286	297
kg	85	90	95	100	105	110	115	120	125	130	140
mL/hr											
70	27.5	25.9	24.6	23.3	22.2	21.2	20.3	19.4	18.7	17.9	16.7
75	29.4	27.6	26.3	25	23.8	22.7	21.8	20.8	20	19.6	17.9
80	31.4	29.6	28.1	26.7	25.4	24.2	23.2	22.2	21.4	20.5	19
85	33.3	31.5	29.8	28.3	27	25.8	24.6	23.6	22.7	21.8	20.2
90	35.3	33.3	31.6	30	28.6	27.3	24.6	25	24	23.1	21.4

Dose (mcg/kg/min) = CF × Rate (mL/hr).

Calculation Factors (CF) by Patient Weight (85-140 kg)

kg	85	90	95	100	105	110	115	120	125	130	140
CF	0.392	0.370	0.351	0.333	0.317	0.303	0.290	0.278	0.267	0.256	0.238

Dopamine (Intropin)

USES

Correction of hemodynamic imbalances present in shock syndrome resulting from myocardial infarction (MI), trauma, septicemia, open heart surgery, renal failure, and chronic cardiac decompensation as in congestive heart failure (CHF).

SOLUTION PREPARATION

Premixed bag: 400 mg dopamine/250 mL D5W.
Final concentration: 1600 mcg/mL.

DOSE

1. **Renal perfusion:** Rates of 1-5 mcg/kg/min are administered.
2. **Hypotension:** An initial dose of 5 mcg/kg/min may be used and increased gradually in 5-10 mcg/kg/min increments up to 20 mcg/kg/min. (Contact physician if 20 mcg/kg/min does not maintain BP.)

WARNINGS

1. Dopamine should not be used in patients with pheochromocytoma.
2. Patients who have been treated with MAO inhibitors (e.g., Marplan, Nardil, or Parnate) will require a reduced starting dose of dopamine—usually at least 1/10 of the usual dose.
3. Avoid cyclopropane or halogenated hydrocarbon anesthetics.
4. Extravasation or peripheral ischemia can cause sloughing and necrosis of tissue in the surrounding area. **Antidote:** The site should be infiltrated with a 10-mL solution containing 5 mg phentolamine (Regitine); a fine hypodermic needle should be used; obtain a physician's order for the antidote.

ADVERSE REACTIONS

Most common are ectopic beats, nausea, vomiting, tachycardia, anginal pain, palpitation, dyspnea, headache, hypotension, and vasoconstriction. Less common are aberrant conduction, bradycardia, piloerection, widening QRS complex, azotemia, and elevated BP.

INCOMPATIBILITY

Acyclovir
Alteplase
Amphotericin B
Ampicillin
Cefazolin
Cefepime
Gentamicin
Imferon

Indomethacin
Insulin
Metronidazole
Penicillin G
Potassium
Sodium bicarbonate
Thiopental

COMPATIBILITY

Alatrofloxacin
Aldesleukin
Amifostine
Aminophylline
Amiodarone
Atracurium
Aztreonam
Bretylium
Cefpirome

Ciprofloxacin
Cisatracurium
Cladribine
Diltiazem
Dobutamine
Docetaxel
Doxorubicin
Enalaprilat
Epinephrine

Esmolol
Etoposide
Famotidine
Fentanyl
Gatifloxacin
Gemcitabine
Granisetron
Haloperidol
Heparin
Hydrocortisone
Hydromorphone
Inamrinone
Labetalol
Levofloxacin
Lidocaine
Linezolid
Lorazepam
Meperidine
Methylprednisolone

Metronidazole
Midazolam
Milrinone
Nitroglycerin
Nitroprusside
Norepinephrine
Ondansetron
Pancuronium
Piperacillin/Tazobactam
Potassium chloride
Propofol
Ranitidine
Streptokinase
Tacrolimus
Theophylline
Vecuronium
Verapamil
Warfarin
Zidovudine

Dopamine (Intropin)

Dopamine (Intropin)

NURSING CONSIDERATIONS

1. An accurate weight should be obtained before administration of dopamine.
2. Consult the Dopamine Drip Rate Calculation Chart to determine the drip rate.
3. Except in cardiac arrest situations, dopamine should be administered via an IV pump to ensure controlled infusion.
4. The *renal perfusion* patient's BP should be monitored and documented hourly. The *hypotensive* patient's BP should be monitored with each increase in dose while dopamine is being incrementally increased. After the desired results are obtained, monitor BP at least hourly and document. Any disproportionate rise or fall in BP should be noted and reported immediately to the physician.
5. Closely document changes in skin color or temperature in the extremities as a monitor for ischemia. Closely document changes in HR, renal output, and signs of reversal of confusion or comatose state as a monitor of drug effectiveness.

Dopamine (Intropin) Drip Rate Calculation Chart—
Patient Weight 35-85 kg (77-189 lbs)
Concentration: 1.6 mg/mL (400 mg/250 mL)

lbs	77	88	99	110	121	132	143	154	165	176	189
kg	35	40	45	50	55	60	65	70	75	80	85
mL/hr	mcg/kg/min										
5	3.8	3.4	2.9	2.6	2.4	2.2	2	1.9	1.8	1.6	1.6
10	7.6	6.7	5.9	5.3	4.9	4.5	4.1	3.8	3.6	3.3	3.1
15	11.4	10	8.9	8	7.3	6.6	6.1	5.7	5.3	5	4.7
20	15.2	13.3	11.8	10.7	9.7	8.9	8.2	7.6	7.1	6.7	6.3
25	19	16.6	14.8	13.4	12.1	11.1	10.2	9.5	8.9	8.4	7.8
30	22.8	20	17.8	16	14.6	13.3	12.3	11.4	10.7	10	9.4
35	26.6	23.3	20.7	18.6	17	15.5	14.3	13.3	12.4	11.6	11
40	30.5	26.7	23.7	21.3	19.4	17.8	16.4	15.2	14.2	13.3	12.3
45	34.3	30	26.6	24	21.8	20	18.4	17.1	16	15	14.1
50	38.1	33.3	29.6	26.7	24.2	22.2	25	19	17.8	16.7	15.7
55	41.9	36.6	32.6	29.3	26.6	24.4	22.5	20.9	19.5	18.3	17.2
60	45.7	40	35.6	32	29.1	26.7	24.6	22.9	21.3	20	18.8
65	49.5	43.4	38.6	34.7	31.6	28.9	26.7	24.8	23.1	21.7	20.4

Continued

Dopamine (Intropin)

Dopamine (Intropin)

Dopamine (Intropin) Drip Rate Calculation Chart—Patient Weight 35-85 kg (77-189 lbs)—cont'd
Concentration: 1.6 mg/mL (400 mg/250 mL)

| lbs | 77 | 88 | 99 | 110 | 121 | 132 | 143 | 154 | 165 | 176 | 189 |
kg	35	40	45	50	55	60	65	70	75	80	85
mL/hr	mcg/kg/min										
70	53.5	46.7	41.5	37.3	34	31.1	28.7	26.7	24.9	23.3	22
75	57.1	50	44.5	40	36.4	33.4	30.8	28.6	26.7	25	23.6
80	60.9	53.3	47.4	42.3	38.8	35.6	32.8	30.5	28.4	26.7	25.1
90	68.6	60	53.3	48	43.6	40	36.9	34.3	32	30	28.7
100	76.2	66.7	59.3	53.3	48.5	44.5	41	38.1	35.6	33.3	31.4

Calculation Factors (CF) for Patient Weight 35-85 kg

kg	35	40	45	50	55	60	65	70	75	80	85
CF	0.762	0.665	0.593	0.533	0.485	0.444	0.410	0.381	0.356	0.333	0.314

Dopamine (Intropin) Drip Rate Calculation Chart—
Patient Weight 90-140 kg (199-297 lbs)
Concentration: 1.6 mg/mL (400 mg/250 mL)

lbs	199	209	220	231	242	253	264	275	286	297
kg	90	95	100	105	110	115	120	125	130	140
mL/hr										
5	1.5	1.4	1.3	1.3	1.2	1.2	1.1	1.1	1	1
10	3	2.8	2.7	2.5	2.4	2.3	2.2	2.1	2	1.9
15	4.4	4.2	4	3.8	3.6	3.5	3.3	3.2	3	2.9
20	5.9	5.6	5.3	5.1	4.9	4.6	4.4	4.3	4.1	3.8
25	7.4	7	6.6	6.3	6	5.8	5.5	5.3	5.1	4.8
30	8.9	8.4	8	7.6	7.3	7	6.6	6.4	6.1	5.7
35	10.3	9.8	9.3	8.9	8.6	8.1	7.7	7.4	7.1	6.7
40	11.9	11.2	10.7	10.2	9.7	9.2	8.8	8.5	8.2	7.6
45	15.3	12.6	12	11.4	10.9	10.4	10	9.6	9.2	8.6
50	14.8	14	13.3	12.7	12.1	11.6	11.1	10.7	10.2	9.5
55	16.3	15.4	14.6	13.9	13.3	12.7	12.3	11.8	11.2	10.5
60	17.8	16.8	16	15.2	14.6	13.9	13.3	12.8	12.3	11.4
65	19.3	18.2	17.4	16.5	15.8	15	14.4	13.9	13.3	12.4

Continued

Dopamine (Intropin)

Dopamine (Intropin)

Dopamine (Intropin) Drip Rate Calculation Chart—
Patient Weight 90-140 kg (199-297 lbs)—cont'd
Concentration: 1.6 mg/mL (400 mg/250 mL)

lbs kg	199 90	209 95	220 100	231 105	242 110	253 115	264 120	275 125	286 130	297 140
mL/hr										
70	20.7	19.6	18.7	17.8	17	16.2	15.5	14.7	14.3	13.3
75	22.2	21.1	20	19.1	18.2	17.3	16.6	16	15.3	14.4
80	23.7	22.5	21.3	23	19.4	18.5	17.7	17.1	16.4	15.2
90	26.7	25.3	24	22.9	21.8	20.8	19.9	19	18.4	17.1
100	29.6	28.1	26.7	25.4	24.3	23.7	22.2	21.3	20.5	19

Dose (mcg/kg/min) = CF × Rate (mL/hr).

Calculation Factors (CF) for Patient Weight 90-140 kg

kg	90	95	100	105	110	115	120	125	130	140
CF	0.296	0.281	0.267	0.254	0.242	0.232	0.222	0.213	0.205	0.190

Drotrecogin Alfa (Xigris)

USES

1. A recombinant form of human activated protein C.
2. Xigris is indicated to reduce mortality in adult patients with severe sepsis associated with acute organ dysfunctions that have a high risk of death.

SOLUTION PREPARATION

1. Reconstitute the 5-mg vials with 2.5 ml sterile water for injection, USP. The 20-mg vials must be reconstituted with 10 mL of sterile water for injection, USP. This results in a concentration of approximately 2 mg/mL. This solution can be held for only 3 hours.
2. The reconstituted solution must be further diluted with sterile 0.9% sodium chloride injection. The IV solution should be prepared immediately after reconstitution in the vials. IV administration must be completed within 12 hours after the IV solution is prepared.

DOSE

See Drotrecogin Dosing Charts. Administer IV at infusion rate of 24 mcg/kg/hr for 96 hours. No dose escalation or bolus is warranted.

CONTRAINDICATIONS

1. Active internal bleed.
2. Hemorrhagic stroke within last 3 months.
3. Platelet count of <30,000.
4. Recent intracranial or intraspinal surgery or severe head trauma requiring hospitalization (in last 2 months); trauma patient with increased risk of life-threatening bleeding.
5. Patients with epidural catheters or within 12 hours of epidural catheter removal.
6. Intracranial neoplasm or mass lesion.
7. Hypersensitivity to drotrecogin or any component of the product.
8. Efficacy has not been established in patients with lower risk of death (APACHE II score <25).

9. Use caution when giving with other anticoagulants or if PTT/PT are elevated.

WARNINGS

1. Therapeutic heparin (>15,000 units/day) or low molecular weight heparin (LMWH).
2. GI bleed within past 6 months.
3. Administration of thrombolytic therapy within past 3 days.
4. Administration of oral anticoagulants or glycoprotein IIb/IIIa inhibitors within past 7 days.
5. Administration of aspirin >650 mg/day or other platelet inhibitors within past 7 days.
6. Ischemic stroke in past 3 months.
7. Intracranial arteriovenous malformation or aneurysm.
8. Known bleeding diathesis except for acute coagulopathy related to sepsis.
9. Chronic severe hepatic disease.
10. Any other condition in which bleeding constitutes a significant hazard.
11. Patients who are pregnant or breastfeeding.

ADVERSE REACTIONS

The most common adverse effect is bleeding.

INCOMPATIBILITY

Administer Xigris through a dedicated IV line or a dedicated lumen in a multilumen central venous catheter. The only solutions Xigris can be administered within the same IV line are as follows: 0.9% sodium chloride, lactated Ringer's, dextrose, or dextrose and saline mixtures.

NURSING CONSIDERATIONS

The aPTT is not reliable for the status of coagulopathy in patients on Xigris, so only the PT is a valuable lab test.

Drotrecogin Alfa (Xigris)

Drotrecogin Alfa (Xigris)

Drotrecogin (Xigris) Dosing Chart
24 mcg/kg/hr for 96 hours
Add 10 mg (2 × 5-mg vials) to 100 mL NS
Final Concentration: 100 mcg/mL

Actual patient weight	Amount of drotrecogin	Concentration	Rate	Approximate time to infuse
40 kg	10 mg	100 mcg/mL	9.6 mL/hr	10 hrs
41 kg	10 mg	100 mcg/mL	9.8 mL/hr	10 hrs
42 kg	10 mg	100 mcg/mL	10.1 mL/hr	10 hrs
43 kg	10 mg	100 mcg/mL	10.3 mL/hr	10 hrs
44 kg	10 mg	100 mcg/mL	10.6 mL/hr	9 hrs
45 kg	10 mg	100 mcg/mL	10.8 mL/hr	9 hrs
46 kg	10 mg	100 mcg/mL	11 mL/hr	9 hrs
47 kg	10 mg	100 mcg/mL	11.3 mL/hr	9 hrs
48 kg	10 mg	100 mcg/mL	11.5 mL/hr	9 hrs
49 kg	10 mg	100 mcg/mL	11.8 mL/hr	9 hrs
50 kg	10 mg	100 mcg/mL	12 mL/hr	8 hrs
51 kg	10 mg	100 mcg/mL	12.2 mL/hr	8 hrs
52 kg	10 mg	100 mcg/mL	12.5 mL/hr	8 hrs
53 kg	10 mg	100 mcg/mL	12.7 mL/hr	8 hrs

54 kg	10 mg	100 mcg/mL	13 mL/hr	8 hrs
55 kg	10 mg	100 mcg/mL	13.2 mL/hr	8 hrs
56 kg	10 mg	100 mcg/mL	13.4 mL/hr	7 hrs
57 kg	10 mg	100 mcg/mL	13.7 mL/hr	7 hrs
58 kg	10 mg	100 mcg/mL	13.9 mL/hr	7 hrs
59 kg	10 mg	100 mcg/mL	14.2 mL/hr	7 hrs
60 kg	10 mg	100 mcg/mL	14.4 mL/hr	7 hrs
61 kg	10 mg	100 mcg/mL	14.6 mL/hr	7 hrs
62 kg	10 mg	100 mcg/mL	14.9 mL/hr	7 hrs
63 kg	10 mg	100 mcg/mL	15.1 mL/hr	7 hrs
64 kg	10 mg	100 mcg/mL	15.4 mL/hr	7 hrs
65 kg	10 mg	100 mcg/mL	15.6 mL/hr	6 hrs
66 kg	10 mg	100 mcg/mL	15.8 mL/hr	6 hrs

Drotrecogin Alfa (Xigris)

Drotrecogin Alfa (Xigris)

Drotrecogin (Xigris) Dosing Chart
24 mcg/kg/hr for 96 hours
Add 20 mg to 100 mL NS
Final Concentration: 200 mcg/mL

Actual patient weight	Amount of drotrecogin	Concentration	Rate	Approximate time to infuse
67 kg	20 mg	200 mcg/mL	8 mL/hr	12 hrs
68 kg	20 mg	200 mcg/mL	8.2 mL/hr	12 hrs
69 kg	20 mg	200 mcg/mL	8.3 mL/hr	12 hrs
70 kg	20 mg	200 mcg/mL	8.4 mL/hr	12 hrs
71 kg	20 mg	200 mcg/mL	8.5 mL/hr	12 hrs
72 kg	20 mg	200 mcg/mL	8.6 mL/hr	12 hrs
73 kg	20 mg	200 mcg/mL	8.8 mL/hr	11 hrs
74 kg	20 mg	200 mcg/mL	8.9 mL/hr	11 hrs
75 kg	20 mg	200 mcg/mL	9 mL/hr	11 hrs
76 kg	20 mg	200 mcg/mL	9.1 mL/hr	11 hrs
77 kg	20 mg	200 mcg/mL	9.2 mL/hr	11 hrs
78 kg	20 mg	200 mcg/mL	9.4 mL/hr	11 hrs
79 kg	20 mg	200 mcg/mL	9.5 mL/hr	11 hrs
80 kg	20 mg	200 mcg/mL	9.6 mL/hr	10 hrs
81 kg	20 mg	200 mcg/mL	9.7 mL/hr	10 hrs

82 kg	20 mg	200 mcg/mL	9.8 mL/hr	10 hrs
83 kg	20 mg	200 mcg/mL	10 mL/hr	10 hrs
84 kg	20 mg	200 mcg/mL	10.1 mL/hr	10 hrs
85 kg	20 mg	200 mcg/mL	10.2 mL/hr	10 hrs
86 kg	20 mg	200 mcg/mL	10.3 mL/hr	10 hrs
87 kg	20 mg	200 mcg/mL	10.4 mL/hr	10 hrs
88 kg	20 mg	200 mcg/mL	10.6 mL/hr	9 hrs
89 kg	20 mg	200 mcg/mL	10.7 mL/hr	9 hrs
90 kg	20 mg	200 mcg/mL	10.8 mL/hr	9 hrs
91 kg	20 mg	200 mcg/mL	10.9 mL/hr	9 hrs
92 kg	20 mg	200 mcg/mL	11 mL/hr	9 hrs
93 kg	20 mg	200 mcg/mL	11.2 mL/hr	9 hrs
94 kg	20 mg	200 mcg/mL	11.3 mL/hr	9 hrs
95 kg	20 mg	200 mcg/mL	11.4 mL/hr	9 hrs
96 kg	20 mg	200 mcg/mL	11.5 mL/hr	9 hrs
97 kg	20 mg	200 mcg/mL	11.6 mL/hr	9 hrs
98 kg	20 mg	200 mcg/mL	11.8 mL/hr	9 hrs
99 kg	20 mg	200 mcg/mL	11.9 mL/hr	8 hrs
100 kg	20 mg	200 mcg/mL	12 mL/hr	8 hrs
101 kg	20 mg	200 mcg/mL	12.1 mL/hr	8 hrs

Continued

Drotrecogin Alfa (Xigris)

Drotrecogin Alfa (Xigris)

Drotrecogin (Xigris) Dosing Chart—cont'd
24 mcg/kg/hr for 96 hours
Add 20 mg to 100 mL NS
Final Concentration: 200 mcg/mL

Actual patient weight	Amount of drotrecogin	Concentration	Rate	Approximate time to infuse
102 kg	20 mg	200 mcg/mL	12.2 mL/hr	8 hrs
103 kg	20 mg	200 mcg/mL	12.4 mL/hr	8 hrs
104 kg	20 mg	200 mcg/mL	12.5 mL/hr	8 hrs
105 kg	20 mg	200 mcg/mL	12.6 mL/hr	8 hrs
106 kg	20 mg	200 mcg/mL	12.7 mL/hr	8 hrs
107 kg	20 mg	200 mcg/mL	12.8 mL/hr	8 hrs
108 kg	20 mg	200 mcg/mL	13 mL/hr	8 hrs
109 kg	20 mg	200 mcg/mL	13.1 mL/hr	8 hrs
110 kg	20 mg	200 mcg/mL	13.2 mL/hr	8 hrs
111 kg	20 mg	200 mcg/mL	13.3 mL/hr	8 hrs
112 kg	20 mg	200 mcg/mL	13.4 mL/hr	7 hrs
113 kg	20 mg	200 mcg/mL	13.6 mL/hr	7 hrs
114 kg	20 mg	200 mcg/mL	13.7 mL/hr	7 hrs
115 kg	20 mg	200 mcg/mL	13.8 mL/hr	7 hrs
116 kg	20 mg	200 mcg/mL	13.9 mL/hr	7 hrs

117 kg	20 mg	200 mcg/mL	14 mL/hr	7 hrs
118 kg	20 mg	200 mcg/mL	14.2 mL/hr	7 hrs
119 kg	20 mg	200 mcg/mL	14.3 mL/hr	7 hrs
120 kg	20 mg	200 mcg/mL	14.4 mL/hr	7 hrs
121 kg	20 mg	200 mcg/mL	14.5 mL/hr	7 hrs
122 kg	20 mg	200 mcg/mL	14.6 mL/hr	7 hrs
123 kg	20 mg	200 mcg/mL	14.8 mL/hr	7 hrs
124 kg	20 mg	200 mcg/mL	14.9 mL/hr	7 hrs
125 kg	20 mg	200 mcg/mL	15 mL/hr	7 hrs
126 kg	20 mg	200 mcg/mL	15.1 mL/hr	7 hrs
127 kg	20 mg	200 mcg/mL	15.2 mL/hr	7 hrs
128 kg	20 mg	200 mcg/mL	15.4 mL/hr	7 hrs
129 kg	20 mg	200 mcg/mL	15.5 mL/hr	6 hrs
130 kg	20 mg	200 mcg/mL	15.6 mL/hr	6 hrs
131 kg	20 mg	200 mcg/mL	15.7 mL/hr	6 hrs
132 kg	20 mg	200 mcg/mL	15.8 mL/hr	6 hrs
133 kg	20 mg	200 mcg/mL	16 mL/hr	6 hrs
134 kg	20 mg	200 mcg/mL	16.1 mL/hr	6 hrs
135 kg	20 mg	200 mcg/mL	16.2 mL/hr	6 hrs

Drotrecogin Alfa (Xigris)

Epinephrine (Adrenalin) Injection

USES
1. Adjunct in the management of cardiac arrest to restore cardiac rhythm.
2. Conversion of fine, low-amplitude fibrillation to a higher amplitude activity before cardioversion.
3. Emergency treatment of severe acute anaphylactic reactions.

SOLUTION PREPARATION
An epinephrine drip is prepared by adding 1 mg epinephrine to 250 mL D5W or NS. **Final concentration:** 1 mg/250 mL (4 mcg/mL).
NOTE: Solutions of double strength (2 mg/250 mL equal to 8 mcg/mL) and triple strength (3 mg/250 mL equal to 12 mcg/mL) also may be prepared.

DOSE
1. Cardiac arrest
   a. As bolus of 1.0 mg IVP, repeat every 3-5 minutes if needed; each dose should be followed by 20 mL NS to ensure drug delivery.
   b. Epinephrine bolus may be given via endotracheal tube or by intracardiac injection if there is difficulty in starting IV.
   c. Epinephrine may be infused as a continuous infusion (after bolus) at a rate of 1-4 mcg/min.
2. Severe anaphylactic reaction
   a. 0.1-0.5 mg SC or IM; if severe anaphylactic shock, give 0.1-0.25 mg slow IVP.
   b. IV bolus may be followed by a continuous infusion at a rate of 1-4 mcg/min, if necessary.

WARNINGS
1. Epinephrine increases myocardia oxygen demand and should not be used in cardiogenic shock.
2. Epinephrine should not be used in traumatic or hemorrhagic shock.
3. Intracardiac epinephrine injection runs the risk of coronary artery laceration, cardiac tamponade, pneumothorax, and intramyocardial injection of the drug.

4. Epinephrine may cause potentially fatal ventricular arrhythmias including fibrillation; use with care in patients with organic heart disease or those receiving other drugs that sensitize the heart.

ADVERSE REACTIONS

1. *Cardiovascular:* Arrhythmias, increased HR, may precipitate angina pectoris, hypertension.
2. May produce a variety of CNS changes.
3. Nausea, vomiting, sweating and respiratory difficulty.

INCOMPATIBILITY

Aminophylline   Thiopental
Sodium bicarbonate

COMPATIBILITY

Atracurium   Dobutamine
Diltiazem   Dopamine

Etomidate   Nitroglycerin
Heparin   Norepinephrine
Inamrinone   Propofol
Labetalol   Potassium chloride
Midazolam

NURSING CONSIDERATIONS

1. Consult the Epinephrine Drip Rate Calculation Chart to determine the drip rate.
2. Except in cardiac arrest situations, epinephrine should be administered via an IV pump to ensure controlled infusion.
3. The patient's BP and HR should be monitored every 2-5 minutes until patient is stabilized, then every 15 minutes.
4. Patient should be closely monitored while receiving IV epinephrine. Document BP and HR; observe and report rate and character (regularity and force) of the pulse.

Epinephrine (Adrenalin) Injection

Epinephrine (Adrenalin) Drip Rate Calculation Chart
Epinephrine 1 mg/250 mL (Concentration: 4 mcg/mL)

Dose	Infusion rate
1 mcg/min	15 mL/hr
1.5 mcg/min	22 mL/hr
2 mcg/min	30 mL/hr
2.5 mcg/min	37 mL/hr
3 mcg/min	45 mL/hr
3.5 mcg/min	52 mL/hr
4 mcg/min	60 mL/hr
5 mcg/min	75 mL/hr
6 mcg/min	90 mL/hr
7 mcg/min	105 mL/hr
8 mcg/min	120 mL/hr

Dose (mcg/kg/min) = CF × Rate (mL/hr).

Calculation Factors (CF) by Patient Weight (40-120 kg)

kg	40	50	60	70	80	90	100	110	120
CF	0.001660	0.001330	0.001110	0.00952	0.00833	0.00740	0.00666	0.00606	0.00555

Double Strength Epinephrine (Adrenalin) Drip Rate Calculation Chart
Epinephrine 2 mg/250 mL (Concentration: 8 mcg/mL)

Dose	Infusion rate
1 mcg/min	7.5 mL/hr
1.5 mcg/min	11 mL/hr
2 mcg/min	15 mL/hr
2.5 mcg/min	19 mL/hr
3 mcg/min	23 mL/hr
3.5 mcg/min	26 mL/hr
4 mcg/min	30 mL/hr
5 mcg/min	38 mL/hr
6 mcg/min	45 mL/hr
7 mcg/min	53 mL/hr
8 mcg/min	60 mL/hr

Dose (mcg/kg/min) = CF $\times$ Rate (mL/hr).

Calculation Factors (CF) 8 mcg/mL by Patient Weight (40-120 kg)

kg	40	50	60	70	80	90	100	110	120
CF	0.00333	0.00266	0.00222	0.00190	0.00166	0.00148	0.00133	0.00121	0.00111

Epinephrine (Adrenalin) Injection

Epinephrine (Adrenalin) Injection

Triple Strength Epinephrine (Adrenalin) Drip Rate Calculation Chart
Epinephrine 3 mg/250 mL (Concentration: 12 mcg/mL)

Dose	Infusion rate
1 mcg/min	5 mL/hr
1.5 mcg/min	7.5 mL/hr
2 mcg/min	10 mL/hr
2.5 mcg/min	13 mL/hr
3 mcg/min	15 mL/hr
3.5 mcg/min	18 mL/hr
4 mcg/min	20 mL/hr
5 mcg/min	25 mL/hr
6 mcg/min	30 mL/hr
7 mcg/min	35 mL/hr
8 mcg/min	40 mL/hr

Dose (mcg/kg/min) = CF $\times$ Rate (mL/hr).

Calculation Factors (CF) for 12 mcg/mL by Patient Weight (40-120 kg)

kg	40	50	60	70	80	90	100	110	120
CF	0.005000	0.004000	0.003330	0.002860	0.002500	0.002220	0.002000	0.001818	0.001666

Eptifibatide (Integrilin)

USES

1. A cyclic heptapeptide antagonist of the platelet glycoprotein (GP) IIb/IIIa receptor, which inhibits platelet aggregation.
2. Integrilin, in combination with heparin, is indicated for the treatment of acute coronary syndromes (e.g., unstable angina, non–Q-wave myocardial infarction [MI]), including those patients who are to be managed medically and those undergoing PTCA.

SOLUTION PREPARATION

1. Obtain the bolus dose from the 10-mL vial containing 20 mg Integrilin (20 mg/10 mL). See the dosing chart.
2. Administer the bolus dose via IV push over 1-2 minutes. Start the continuous infusion undiluted from the 75-mg/100-mL vial. Use vented tubing. Solution is good for 24 hours.

DOSE

1. *Acute coronary syndrome:* The recommended dose for patients with normal renal function (i.e., creatinine <2) is 180 mcg/kg bolus as soon as possible, followed by 2 mcg/kg/min infusion up to the time of discharge, CABG surgery, or 72 hours. For patients with renal insufficiency (i.e., creatinine 2-4), use 180 mcg/kg bolus and 1 mcg/kg/min infusion.
2. *Percutaneous coronary intervention (PCI):* The recommended dose for patients with normal renal function (i.e., creatinine <2) is 180 mcg/kg bolus and 2.0 mcg/kg/min infusion. A second bolus of 180 mcg/kg is given 10 minutes after the first bolus. For patients with renal insufficiency (i.e., creatinine 2-4), use 180-mcg/kg bolus and a 1 mcg/kg/min infusion. A second bolus of 180 mcg/kg is repeated after the first bolus.

WARNINGS

1. Bleeding is the most common complication encountered during therapy with eptifibatide.

2. Use with caution in patients with platelet count <150,000/mm^3
3. Use with caution in patients with hemorrhagic retinopathy.
4. Caution should be employed when using with other drugs that affect hemostasis.
5. During therapy with eptifibatide, patients should be monitored for potential bleeding. When bleeding cannot be controlled with pressure, infusion of eptifibatide and heparin should be discontinued.

ADVERSE REACTIONS

The most common adverse effect is bleeding.

INCOMPATIBILITY

Furosemide

COMPATIBILITY

Alteplase (tPA)	Dextrose 5% NS
Atropine	Dobutamine
Heparin	Nitroglycerin
Lidocaine	Normal saline
Meperidine	Potassium chloride
Metoprolol	(up to 60 mEq)
Midazolam	Verapamil
Morphine	

NURSING CONSIDERATIONS

1. Check the patient's ACT, aPTT, and platelet count at baseline; check again within 6 hours after loading infusion, and check at least daily thereafter during therapy.
2. If patient experiences a platelet decrease to <90,000/mm^3, additional platelet counts should be performed to exclude pseudothrombocytopenia. If thrombocytopenia is confirmed, eptifibatide and heparin should be discontinued.
3. In PTCA, before pulling the sheath, heparin should be discontinued for 3-4 hours; ACT <180 seconds or PTT <45 seconds should be documented.

Eptifibatide (Integrilin)

Eptifibatide (Integrilin)

Eptifibatide (Integrilin) Dosing Chart
ESPRIT Trial Dosing for PCI: 180-mcg/kg Bolus, Then 2 mcg/kg/min Infusion, Followed by a Second 180-mcg/kg Bolus 10 Minutes After the First Bolus—Normal Renal Function (Creatinine <2)

Patient weight (kg)	First bolus dose (mL): use 20-mg/10-mL vial	Maintenance dose (mL/hr): use 75-mg/100-mL premixed vial	Second bolus dose (mL): use 20-mg/10-mL vial
42-46	4	7	4
47-53	4.5	8	4.5
54-59	5	9	5
60-65	5.6	10	5.6
66-71	6.2	11	6.2
72-78	6.8	12	6.8
79-84	7.3	13	7.3
85-90	7.9	14	7.9
91-96	8.5	15	8.5
97-103	9	16	9
104-109	9.5	17	9.5
110-115	10.2	18	10.2
116-121	10.7	19	10.7
>121	11.3	20	11.3

Eptifibatide (Integrilin) Dosing Chart

ESPRIT Trial Dosing for PCI: 180-mcg/kg Bolus, Then 1 mcg/kg/min Infusion, Followed by a Second 180-mcg/kg Bolus 10 Minutes After the First Bolus—Reduced Renal Function (Creatinine 2-4)

Patient weight (kg)	First bolus dose (mL): use 20-mg/10-mL vial	Maintenance dose (mL/hr): use 75-mg/100-mL premixed vial	Second bolus dose (mL): use 20-mg/10-mL vial
42-46	4	3.5	4
47-53	4.5	4	4.5
54-59	5	4.5	5
60-65	5.6	5	5.6
66-71	6.2	5.5	6.2
72-78	6.8	6	6.8
79-84	7.3	6.5	7.3
85-90	7.9	7	7.9
91-96	8.5	7.5	8.5
97-103	9	8	9
104-109	9.5	8.5	9.5
110-115	10.2	9	10.2
116-121	10.7	9.5	10.7
>121	11.3	10	11.3

Eptifibatide (Integrilin)

Eptifibatide (Integrilin)

Eptifibatide (Integrilin) Dosing Chart
ESPRIT Trial Dosing: 180-mcg/kg Bolus, Then 0.5-mcg/kg/min Infusion, Followed by a Second 180-mcg/kg Bolus 10 Minutes After the First Bolus—Patients at High Risk for Bleeding

Patient weight (kg)	First bolus dose (mL): use 20-mg/10-mL vial	Maintenance dose (mL/hr): use 75-mg/100-mL premixed vial	Second bolus dose (mL): use 20-mg/10-mL vial
42-46	4	2	4
47-53	4.5	2	4.5
54-59	5	2.3	5
60-65	5.6	2.5	5.6
66-71	6.2	2.7	6.2
72-78	6.8	3	6.8
79-84	7.3	3.2	7.3
85-90	7.9	3.5	7.9
91-96	8.5	3.7	8.5
97-103	9	4	9
104-109	9.5	4.3	9.5
110-115	10.2	4.5	10.2
>116	10.5	5	10.5

Esmolol (Brevibloc)

USES

1. Treatment of supraventricular tachycardia, atrial fibrillation, or flutter (primarily to control ventricular rate). Esmolol is a short-acting beta-blocker.
2. Control of BP in perioperative hypertension.

SOLUTION PREPARATION

Mix 2.5 g esmolol (10 mL of 250-mg/mL vial) in 250 mL D5W or NS. **Final concentration:** 10 mg/mL. Stable for 24 hours.

DOSE

The usual loading dose is 500 mcg/kg/min over 1 minute, followed by infusion of 50-mcg/kg/min infusion for 4 minutes. If response is inadequate, repeat bolus 500 mcg/kg over 1 minute and increase infusion to 100 mcg/kg/min. Maximum recommended maintenance infusion is 200 mcg/kg/min. Usual dose range is 50-200 mcg/kg/min and average dose is 100 mcg/kg/min.

WARNINGS

1. Esmolol is contraindicated in patients with sinus bradycardia or heart block, uncompensated congestive heart failure (CHF), cardiogenic shock, or allergy to beta-blockers.
2. Esmolol should be used with caution in patients with hyperreactive airways, diabetes, hypoglycemia, or renal failure.
3. Esmolol should be administered carefully to avoid extravasation.

ADVERSE REACTIONS

1. *Incidence >10%:* Hypotension, diaphoresis.
2. *Incidence 1%-10%:* Peripheral ischemia, dizziness, somnolence, confusion, headache, agitation, fatigue, nausea, vomiting, infusion site reactions.

INCOMPATIBILITY

Amphotericin B   Warfarin
Furosemide

COMPATIBILITY

Amikacin
Aminophylline
Amiodarone
Ampicillin
Atracurium
Bretylium
Butorphanol
Calcium chloride
Cefazolin
Ceftazidime
Chloramphenicol
Cimetidine
Cisatracurium
Clindamycin
Diltiazem
Dopamine
Enalaprilat
Erythromycin

Famotidine
Fentanyl
Gatifloxacin
Gentamicin
Heparin
Hydrocortisone
Insulin
Labetalol
Linezolid
Magnesium sulfate
Methyldopa
Metronidazole
Midazolam
Morphine
Nafcillin
Nitroglycerin
Nitroprusside
Norepinephrine

Pancuronium
Penicillin G
Phenytoin
Piperacillin
Polymyxin B
Potassium chloride
Potassium phosphate
Propofol

Ranitidine
Remifentanil
Sodium acetate
Streptomycin
Tacrolimus
Trimethoprim/sulfa
Vancomycin
Vecuronium

NURSING CONSIDERATIONS

1. Consult the Esmolol Drip Rate Chart to determine the drip rate.
2. Esmolol should be administered via an IV pump to ensure controlled infusion.
3. The patient's BP, HR, mean arterial pressure (MAP), ECG, and respiratory rate (RR) should be monitored while on therapy.
4. *Drug interaction:* Increased serum digoxin levels.

Esmolol (Brevibloc)

Esmolol (Brevibloc)

Esmolol (Brevibloc) Drip Rate Calculation Chart
Brevibloc 2.5 g in 250 mL (Concentration: 10 mg/mL)

Patient weight		Drip rate			
lbs	kg	50 mcg/kg	100 mcg/kg	150 mcg/kg	200 mcg/kg
110	50	15 mL/hr	30 mL/hr	45 mL/hr	60 mL/hr
132	60	18 mL/hr	36 mL/hr	54 mL/hr	72 mL/hr
154	70	21 mL/hr	42 mL/hr	63 mL/hr	84 mL/hr
176	80	24 mL/hr	48 mL/hr	72 mL/hr	96 mL/hr
198	90	27 mL/hr	54 mL/hr	81 mL/hr	108 mL/hr
220	100	30 mL/hr	60 mL/hr	90 mL/hr	120 mL/hr

Fenoldopam (Corlopam)

USES

Treatment of severe hypertension and in patients with renal compromise; potential use for congestive heart failure (CHF).

SOLUTION PREPARATION

The Corlopam injection ampule must be diluted in 0.9% sodium chloride injection USP or 5% dextrose injection USP using the following dilution schedule: 1 mL (10 mg) added to 250 mL = final concentration of 40 mcg/mL.

DOSE

1. *Severe hypertension:* Initial, 0.1 mcg/kg/min; may be increased in increments of 0.05-0.2 mcg/kg/min until target BP is achieved; average rate, 0.25-0.5 mcg/kg/min; usual length of treatment is 1-6 hours with tapering of 12% every 15-30 minutes.
2. *Renal perfusion:* Initial, 0.05 mcg/kg/min infusion; titrate to a maximum renal perfusion range of 0.1-0.3 mcg/kg/min.

WARNINGS

Use with caution in patients with cirrhosis, portal hypertension (due to possible increase in portal venous pressure), unstable angina, or glaucoma.

ADVERSE REACTIONS

1. *Cardiovascular:* Hypotension, edema, tachycardia, facial flushing, asymptomatic T-wave flattening, flutter (atrial), chest pain, angina in patients with history of unstable angina.
2. *CNS:* Headache, dizziness.
3. *GI:* Nausea, vomiting, diarrhea, xerostomia.
4. *Ocular:* Intraocular pressure (increased), blurred vision.
5. *Other:* Increases in portal pressure in cirrhotic patients.
6. The most common side effects are headache, flushing, nausea, and hypotension, each reported in more than 5% of patients.

DRUG INTERACTIONS

Concurrent acetaminophen may increase fenoldopam levels (30%-90%).

INCOMPATIBILITY

In-line incompatibility: Alkaline solutions (e.g., sodium bicarbonate), furosemide.

COMPATIBILITY

In-line compatibility: Cefazolin, dopamine, epinephrine, gentamicin, heparin, lidocaine, and nitroprusside.

NURSING CONSIDERATIONS

1. Monitor BP, HR, ECG, renal/hepatic function.
2. No known contraindications.
3. No toxic metabolites.
4. Corlopam contains sodium metabisulfite, which may cause allergic-type reactions, including anaphylactic symptoms, in susceptible people. Corlopam also may cause tachycardia, hypokalemia, or an increase in intraocular pressure.

Fenoldopam (Corlopam)

Fenoldopam (Corlopam) Drip Rate Calculation Chart
Infusion Rates (mL/hr) to Achieve a Given Drug Dose Rate (mcg/kg/min)
10 mg in 250 mL (Concentration: 40 mcg/mL)

Patient weight (kg)	Dose rate = 0.05 mcg/kg/min	Dose rate = 0.1 mcg/kg/min	Dose rate = 0.2 mcg/kg/min	Dose rate = 0.3 mcg/kg/min
40	3	6	12	18
50	3.75	7.5	15	22.5
60	4.50	9	18	27
70	5.25	10.5	21	31.5
80	6	12	24	36
90	6.75	13.5	27	40.5
100	7.50	15	30	45
110	8.25	16.5	33	49.5
120	9	18	36	54

Dose (mcg/kg/min) = CF × Rate (mL/hr).

Calculation Factors (CF) by Patient Weight (40-120 kg)

kg	40	50	60	70	80	90	100	110	120
CF	0.0166	0.0133	0.0111	0.0095	0.0083	0.0074	0.0066	0.0060	0.0055

Haloperidol (Haldol)

USES

For rapid tranquilization of the agitated ICU/cardiac care unit (CCU) patient, haloperidol may be administered IV.

SOLUTION PREPARATION

Haldol may be administered by IV push. Haldol is available as 5 mg/mL in 1-mL and 10-mL vials.

DOSE

1. The usual initial dose is 0.5-2 mg IV for mild agitation, 5-10 mg IV for moderate agitation, and 10+ mg for severe agitation.
2. *For subsequent doses:* Double the previous dose every 15-30 minutes until the agitation is resolved.
3. When sedation is achieved, maintain the patient by repeating the last dose at 30-minute intervals PRN.
4. *Maximum dose:* 50-100 mg Haldol given alone or 20 mg Haldol with 1 mg lorazepam (Ativan) IV.
5. *Maximum daily dose:* Up to 480 mg IV per day.

WARNINGS

1. Haldol should not be administered to patients with alcohol or barbiturate withdrawal or brain injury in the past 3-4 days.
2. Contraindicated in patients with narrow angle glaucoma and parkinsonism.
3. Use with caution in patients with cardiovascular disease, seizures, hypotension, CNS depression, or severe liver disease.

ADVERSE REACTIONS

1. Extrapyramidal symptoms, laryngospasm, hypotension, and dysrhythmias.
2. Respiratory depression (enhanced if lorazepam also used).

INCOMPATIBILITY

Heparin   Procainamide
Nitroprusside

COMPATIBILITY

Dobutamine   Midazolam
Dopamine   Nitroglycerin
Lidocaine   Theophylline

NURSING CONSIDERATIONS

1. Observe the patient for onset of drug action 5-30 minutes after the dose is administered.
2. Observe the patient for possible side effects: Laryngospasm—treat with epinephrine 0.1-0.25 mg or 1-2.5 mL IV slowly (keep syringe available at bedside, 1:10,000 concentration, 10 mL syringe); treat extrapyramidal effects with Benadryl IV.
3. The patient's BP should be monitored closely to observe for hypotension.
4. Cardiac arrhythmias may be treated with IV lidocaine.

Haloperidol (Haldol)

Heparin

USES

1. Prophylaxis and treatment of venous thrombosis and its extension; pulmonary embolism, peripheral arterial embolism, atrial fibrillation with embolization.
2. Diagnosis and treatment of acute and chronic consumption coagulopathies (disseminated intravascular coagulation [DIC]).
3. As an adjunct in the treatment of coronary occlusion with acute myocardial infarction (AMI).

SOLUTION PREPARATION

Heparin infusions are available as premixed solutions containing 25,000 units/500 mL D5W (50 units/mL)

DOSE

Dose must be individualized and adjusted according to coagulation tests (PTT). *Usual dosage:* 5000 units loading dose followed by a continuous infusion of 800-1600 units/hr. Monitor PTT every 6 hours early in infusion and adjust infusion rate as needed. Dose is adequate when PTT is 1.5-2 times control. See the weight-based dosing chart.

WARNINGS

1. Hemorrhage can occur at virtually any site in patients receiving heparin. An unexplained fall in hematocrit, fall in BP, or any other unexplained symptom should lead to serious consideration of a hemorrhagic event.
2. Use heparin with extreme caution in disease states in which there is increased danger of hemorrhage (e.g., dissecting aneurysm, increased capillary permeability, severe hypertension, spinal anesthesia, GI ulceration, diverticulitis or ulcerative colitis, and liver disease with impaired hemostasis).
3. Thrombocytopenia may occur in patients receiving heparin; baseline and regular platelet monitoring is recommended.

ADVERSE REACTIONS

1. *Hemorrhage:* Bleeding can usually be controlled by withdrawing the drug. NOTE: 1 mg of protamine will neutralize 100 units of heparin.
2. *Hypersensitivity:* Chills, fever, urticaria and rarely asthma, nausea/vomiting, shock or anaphylactoid reactions.
3. *Thrombocytopenia:* May occur 2-12 days after therapy is begun; platelet counts should be done on a regular basis while patient is receiving heparin infusion.
4. *Other:* Cutaneous necrosis, vasospastic reactions with pain, ischemia and cyanosis in affected limb, suppressed aldosterone synthesis.

INCOMPATIBILITY

Alatrofloxacin
Alteplase
Amikacin
Amiodarone
Amphotericin B
Amsacrine
Ciprofloxacin
Codeine phosphate
Diazepam
Dilantin
Dobutamine
Doxycycline
Ergotamine
Filgrastim
Gatifloxacin
Gentamicin
Haloperidol
Levofloxacin
Methadone
Nicardipine
Phenergan
Tobramycin
Vancomycin

COMPATIBILITY

Acyclovir
Aldesleukin
Allopurinol
Amifostine
Aminophylline
Ampicillin
Ampicillin/sulbactam
Atracurium
Atropine
Aztreonam
Betamethasone
Bleomycin
Calcium gluconate
Cefazolin
Cefotetan
Ceftazidime
Ceftriaxone
Chlordiazepoxide
Chlorpromazine
Cimetidine
Cisplatin
Cladribine
Clindamycin
Cyanocobalamin

Heparin

Cyclophosphamide
Cytarabine
Dexamethasone
Digoxin
Diltiazem
Diphenhydramine
Docetaxel
Dopamine
Doxorubicin
Edrophonium
Enalaprilat
Epinephrine
Erythromycin
Esmolol
Ethacrynate
Etoposide
Famotidine
Fentanyl
Fluconazole
Fludarabine
Fluorouracil
Foscarnet

Furosemide
Gemcitabine
Granisetron
Hydralazine
Hydrocortisone
Hydromorphone
Isoproterenol
Insulin
Kanamycin
Leucovorin
Lidocaine
Linezolid
Lorazepam
Magnesium sulfate
Meperidine
Meropenem
Methotrexate
Methyldopa
Metoclopramide
Metronidazole
Midazolam
Milrinone

Minocycline
Mitomycin
Morphine
Nafcillin
Neostigmine
Nitroglycerin
Nitroprusside
Norepinephrine
Ondansetron
Oxacillin
Oxytocin
Paclitaxel

Pancuronium
Penicillin G
Pentazocine
Piperacillin
Potassium chloride
Procainamide
Prochlorperazine
Theophylline
Vinblastine
Vincristine
Zidovudine

NURSING CONSIDERATIONS

1. Consult the Heparin Drip Rate Calculation Chart to determine drip rate.
2. Heparin should be administered via an IV pump to ensure controlled infusion.
3. Monitor patients for signs/symptoms of hemorrhage; contact physician if symptoms occur.
4. Avoid IM injections.

Heparin Drip Rate Calculation Chart
Heparin 25,000 units/500 mL (Concentration: 50 units/mL)

Dose	Infusion rate
800 units/hr	16 mL/hr
900 units/hr	18 mL/hr
1000 units/hr	20 mL/hr
1100 units/hr	22 mL/hr
1200 units/hr	24 mL/hr
1300 units/hr	26 mL/hr
1400 units/hr	28 mL/hr
1500 units/hr	30 mL/hr
1600 units/hr	32 mL/hr

Heparin

Heparin

Heparin Weight-Based Dosing Protocol
Target PTT: 55-80 Seconds

PTT	Bolus dose	Stop drip	Rate change	Repeat PTT
<40 sec	80 units/kg	0 min	Increase 4 units/kg/hr	6 hr
40-54 sec	40 units/kg	0 min	Increase 2 units/kg/hr	6 hr
55-80 sec	None	0 min	No change	Next AM
81-100 sec	0	30 min	Decrease 2 units/kg/hr	6 hr
>100 sec	0	60 min	Decrease 3 units/kg/hr	6 hr

Patient weight (kg)	Heparin bolus (units; rounded to the nearest 500 units) 80 units/kg (mL)	Initial drip rate 18 units/kg (mL/hr)	40 units/kg (mL)	aPPT dosing adjustments heparin drip rates (units/hr; rounded to the nearest 50 units) Increase 4 units/kg/hr	±2 units/kg/hr	Decrease 3 units/kg/hr
40	3000 (0.6)	750 (15)	1500 (0.3)	150	100	100
45	3500 (0.7)	800 (16)	2000 (0.4)	200	100	150
50	4000 (0.8)	900 (18)	2000 (0.4)	200	100	150
55	4500 (0.9)	1000 (20)	2000 (0.4)	200	100	150

60	5000 (1)	1100 (22)	2500 (0.5)	250	100	200
65	5000 (1)	1150 (23)	2500 (0.5)	250	150	200
70	5500 (1.1)	1250 (25)	3000 (0.6)	300	150	200
75	6000 (1.2)	1350 (27)	3000 (0.6)	300	150	200
80	6500 (1.3)	1450 (29)	3000 (0.6)	300	150	250
85	7000 (1.4)	1550 (31)	3500 (0.7)	350	150	250
90	7000 (1.4)	1600 (32)	3500 (0.7)	350	200	300
95	7500 (1.5)	1700 (34)	4000 (0.8)	400	200	300
100	8000 (1.6)	1800 (36)	4000 (0.8)	400	200	300
105	8500 (1.7)	1900 (38)	4000 (0.8)	400	200	300
110	9000 (1.8)	2000 (40)	4500 (0.9)	450	200	350
115	9000 (1.8)	2050 (41)	4500 (0.9)	450	250	350
120	9500 (1.9)	2150 (43)	5000 (1)	500	250	350
125	10000 (2)	2250 (45)	5000 (1)	500	250	350
130	10000 (2)	2350 (47)	5000 (1)	500	250	400

Heparin

Ideal Body Weight Chart

Height	Males (kg)	Females (kg)
5'0"	50	45.5
5'1"	52.3	47.8
5'2"	54.6	50
5'3"	56.9	52.4
5'4"	59.2	54.7
5'5"	61.5	57
5'6"	63.8	59.3
5'7"	66.1	61.6
5'8"	68.4	63.9
5'9"	70.7	66.2
5'10"	73	68.5
5'11"	75.3	70.8
6'0"	77.6	73.1
6'1"	80	75.4
6'2"	82.2	77.7
6'3"	84.5	80
6'4"	86.8	
6'5"	89.1	
6'6"	91.4	

Ibutilide (Corvert)

USES
Acute termination of atrial fibrillation or flutter; class III antiarrhythmic agent.

SOLUTION PREPARATION
A Corvert infusion is prepared by adding 1 mg (10-mL vial) Corvert to 50 mL D5W or NS. Infuse over 10 minutes (300 mL/hr). If arrhythmia does not terminate in 10 minutes, repeat a second infusion over 10 minutes. May also be given undiluted over 10 minutes.

DOSE
1. For patients weighing ≥60 kg, give 1 mg over 10 minutes.
2. For patients weighing ≤60 kg, give 0.01 mg/kg over 10 minutes.

WARNINGS
1. Observe patients with continuous ECG monitor for at least 4 hours after infusion.
2. Potentially fatal arrhythmias (e.g., ventricular tachycardia), usually in association with torsades de pointes (QT prolongation), may occur with ibutilide (up to 1.7% incidence of arrhythmias in treated patients).

ADVERSE REACTIONS
1. Ventricular tachycardia (2.7%), torsades de pointes (1.7%), ventricular extrasystoles (5.1%), tachycardia/supraventricular tachycardia, hypotension (2%), bundle branch block (1.9%), AV block (1.5%).
2. Headache (3.6%).
3. Nausea (>1%).

INCOMPATIBILITY/INTERACTIONS

1. Avoid use with other antiarrhythmic agents (disopyramide, quinidine, and procainamide) due to increased toxicity. Also, amiodarone and sotalol should be avoided due to their potential to prolong refractoriness.
2. Avoid use with phenothiazines, tricyclic and tetracyclic antidepressants, and nonsedating antihistamines (astemizole) due to QT prolongation.

NURSING CONSIDERATIONS

1. Discontinue infusion if ventricular tachycardia or prolongation of QT occurs.
2. Ibutilide will usually not affect cardiac output, mean pulmonary arterial pressure, or pulmonary capillary wedge pressure (PCWP).
3. Hypokalemia and hypomagnesemia should be corrected prior to use since prolonged QT and arrhythmias are more common.

Immune Globulin Intravenous
(Carimune, Gamimune, Gammagard, Gammar-P, Iveegam, Panglobulin, Polygam, Sandoglobulin, Venoglobulin-S)

USES
For treatment of immunodeficiency syndromes (e.g., hypogammaglobulinemia, agammaglobulinemia), idiopathic thrombocytopenic purpura (ITP), chronic lymphocytic leukemia (CLL), refractory dermatomyositis or polymyositis, autoimmune diseases (e.g., myasthenia gravis or severe rheumatoid arthritis), and Guillain-Barré syndrome.

SOLUTION PREPARATION
Each product requires specific handling. Some products are supplied in ready-to-use form in glass bottles. Lyophilized powder products require the addition of sterile water as the diluent to reconstitute the product. Gently swirl, do not shake, to facilitate reconstitution.

DOSE
1. *Chronic lymphocytic leukemia (CLL):* 400 mg/kg/dose every 3 weeks.
2. *Immunodeficiency disorders:* 200-400 mg/kg every 4 weeks.
3. *ITP:* 400 mg/kg/day for 2-5 days.
4. *Guillain-Barré syndrome:* 400 mg/kg/day for 4 days.
5. *Refractory dermatomyositis:* 2 g/kg/dose monthly.
6. Many additional regimens are published.

WARNINGS
Administer the initial dose slowly. Anaphylactic reactions are possible.

ADVERSE REACTIONS
1. Tachycardia, flushing, nausea, dyspnea.
2. Chills.
3. Anaphylactic reactions.
4. Renal dysfunction, acute renal failure.

INCOMPATIBILITY
Unknown.

COMPATIBILITY
None. Administer via a separate IV line with no other medications.

NURSING CONSIDERATIONS
1. Monitor the patient closely for signs of anaphylaxis during the initial dose and at the beginning of the infusion.
2. Consult the Immune Globulin Drip Rate Calculation Chart to determine the drip rate.
3. Use caution in the elderly and in patients with diabetes, preexisting renal disease, or volume depletion. To minimize risk of renal dysfunction, administer at the lowest rate of infusion and lowest concentration that is practical.

Immune Globulin Intravenous (Carimune, Gamimune, Gammagard, Gammar-P, Iveegam, Panglobulin, Polygam, Sandoglobulin, Venoglobulin-S)

145

Immune Globulin Intravenous

(Carimune, Gamimune, Gammagard, Gammar-P, Iveegam, Panglobulin, Polygam, Sandoglobulin, Venoglobulin-S)

Immune Globulin Drip Rate Calculation Chart

Drug	Available	50-kg doses	60-kg doses	70-kg doses	80-kg doses
Gammar-P	5 g/100 mL	Infuse 30 mL/hr for 15-30 min, increase to 60 mL/hr after 15-30 min, to 90 mL/hr up to a max of 180 mL/hr	Infuse 36 mL/hr for 15-30 min, increase to 72 mL/hr after 15-30 min, to 108 mL/hr to a max of 216 mL/hr	Infuse 42 mL/hr for 15-30 min, increase to 84 mL/hr after 15-30 min, to 126 mL/hr to a max of 252 mL/hr	Infuse 48 mL/hr for 15-30 min, increase to 96 mL/hr after 15-30 min, to 144 mL/hr to a max of 288 mL/hr
Gamimune	5 g/100 mL	Same as Gammar-P	Same as Gammar-P	Same as Gammar-P	Same as Gammar-P
Sandoglobulin	6 g/100 mL	6% solution with initial rate of 60-90 mL/hr increasing after 15-30 min to a max of 150 mL/hr	6% solution with initial rate of 60-90 mL/hr increasing after 15-30 min to a max of 150 mL/hr	6% solution with initial rate of 60-90 mL/hr increasing after 15-30 min to a max of 150 mL/hr	6% solution with initial rate of 60-90 mL/hr increasing after 15-30 min to a max of 150 mL/hr
Carimune	6 g/100 mL*				

Gammagard	5 g/100 mL	Initial 25 mL/hr; if rate causes no patient distress, may gradually increase; not to exceed a max of 200 mL/hr	Initial 30 mL/hr; if rate causes no patient distress, may gradually increase; not to exceed a max of 240 mL/hr	Initial 35 mL/hr; if rate causes no patient distress, may gradually increase; not to exceed a max of 280 mL/hr	Initial 40 mL/hr; if rate causes no patient distress, may gradually increase; not to exceed a max of 320 mL/hr
Polygam	5 g/100 mL	Same as Gammagard	Same as Gammagard	Same as Gammagard	Same as Gammagard

*6 g/200 mL for initial doses to prevent reactions (3% solution).

Immune Globulin Intravenous (Carimune, Gamimune, Gammagard, Gammar-P, Iveegam, Panglobulin, Polygam, Sandoglobulin, Venoglobulin-S)

147

Inamrinone (Inocor)

Previously known as amrinone; name changed to avoid confusion with amiodarone.

USES

For short-term treatment of severe congestive heart failure (CHF) in patients who have not responded adequately to digitalis, diuretics, and/or vasodilators. Its mechanism of action is via its positive inotropic and vasodilatory effects.

SOLUTION PREPARATION

An inamrinone drip is prepared by adding 500 mg (5×100-mg ampules) inamrinone directly to 100 mL 0.9% NaCl. **Final concentration:** 500 mg/200 mL or 2.5 mg/mL. Do not withdraw fluid from the IV bag to compensate for the volume of inamrinone added. Inamrinone may not be added to dextrose-containing solutions; however, it may be piggybacked into a running dextrose infusion.

DOSE

1. Initial bolus of 0.75 mg/kg given slowly over 2-3 minutes; may be repeated in 30 minutes if necessary.
2. Maintenance infusion between 5-10 mcg/kg/min.
3. Total daily dose, including boluses and cumulative infused dose, usually should not exceed 10 mg/kg. (Higher doses, up to 18 mg/kg/day, have been used in a limited number of patients.)

WARNINGS

1. May aggravate symptoms of idiopathic hypertrophic subaortic stenosis.
2. Patients who have received large doses of diuretics may require cautious administration of fluids and electrolytes to ensure sufficient cardiac filling pressure for Inocor to be effective.
3. Inamrinone-induced increases in cardiac output, with resulting diuresis, may require a dose reduction of diuretics to prevent excessive potassium loss.

4. Inamrinone is not recommended for patients with acute myocardial infarction (AMI).
5. *Contraindications:* Patients sensitive to bisulfates (e.g., asthmatics).
6. Increased plasma concentrations of inamrinone may occur in patients with compromised liver or renal function.
7. Excessive hypotension has occurred when used concomitantly with disopyramide (Norpace).

ADVERSE REACTIONS
1. *Thrombocytopenia:* Appears to be dose dependent; consider dosage reduction or discontinue inamrinone.
2. Cardiac arrhythmias.
3. Hypotension.
4. May increase AV conduction.
5. *GI:* Disturbances.
6. *Hepatotoxicity:* Manifested by elevations in liver function tests and clinical symptoms suggestive of idiosyncratic hypersensitivity reaction.

7. Hypersensitivity reactions (e.g., pericarditis, pleuritis, ascites, jaundice, myositis, vasculitis).

INCOMPATIBILITY
Dextrose solutions
Furosemide (Lasix)
Procainamide
Sodium bicarbonate

COMPATIBILITY
Aminophylline
Atropine
Bretylium
Calcium chloride
Cimetidine
Cisatracurium
Digoxin
Dobutamine
Dopamine
Epinephrine
Famotidine
Hydrocortisone
Isoproterenol
Lidocaine
Methylprednisolone
Nitroglycerin
Nitroprusside
Norepinephrine
Phenylephrine
Potassium chloride
Propofol

Inamrinone (Inocor)

NURSING CONSIDERATIONS

1. Depending on the patient's status, an accurate weight should be obtained before the administration of inamrinone.
2. Consult the Inamrinone Drip Rate Calculation Chart to determine the drip rate.
3. Except in cardiac arrest situations, inamrinone should be administered via an IV pump to ensure controlled infusion.
4. BP should be measured every 15 minutes until stable, then at least every hour as long as drip remains in use.
5. Physician should order platelet count before inamrinone administration and daily thereafter.
6. Closely monitor and document changes in central venous pressure (CVP), HR, urine output, body weight, and clinical signs and symptoms of CHF (e.g., orthopnea, dyspnea, fatigue).

Inamrinone (Inocor) Drip Rate Calculation Chart—
Patient Weight 40-75 kg (88-165 lbs)
Concentration: 2.5 mg/mL (500 mg/200 mL Total Volume)

| lbs | 88 | 99 | 110 | 121 | 132 | 143 | 154 | 165 |
kg	40	45	50	55	60	65	70	75
mL/hr								
5	5.2	4.6	4.2	3.8	3.5	3.2	3	2.8
6	6.2	5.6	5	4.5	4.2	3.8	3.6	3.3
7	7.3	6.5	5.8	5.3	4.9	4.5	4.2	3.9
8	8.3	7.4	6.7	6.1	5.6	5.1	4.8	4.4
9	9.4	8.3	7.5	6.8	6.2	5.6	5.4	5
10	10.4	9.3	8.3	7.6	6.9	6.4	6	5.6
15	15.6	13.9	12.5	11.4	10.4	9.6	8.9	8.3
20	20.8	18.5	16.7	15.2	13.9	12.8	11.9	11.1
25	26	23.1	20.8	18.9	17.4	16	14.9	13.9
30	31.2	27.8	25	22.7	20.8	19.2	17.9	16.7

Inamrinone (Inocor)

Inamrinone (Inocor)

Dose (mcg/kg/min) = CF × Rate (mL/hr).

Calculation Factors (CF) by Patient Weight (40-75 kg)

kg	40	45	50	55	60	65	70	75
CF	1.04	0.926	0.833	0.758	0.694	0.641	0.595	0.556

Inamrinone (Inocor) Drip Rate Calculation Chart—
Patient Weight 80-120 kg (176-264 lbs)
Concentration: 2.5 mg/mL (500 mg/200 mL Total Volume)

lbs	176	187	198	209	220	231	242	253	264
kg	80	85	90	95	100	105	110	115	120
mL/hr									
5	2.6	2.4	2.3	2.2	2.1	2	1.9	1.8	1.7
6	3.1	2.9	2.8	2.6	2.5	2.4	2.3	2.2	2.1
7	3.6	3.4	3.2	3.1	2.9	2.8	2.6	2.5	2.4
8	4.2	3.9	3.7	3.5	3.3	3.2	3	2.9	2.8
9	4.7	4.4	4.2	3.9	3.8	3.6	3.4	3.3	3.1
10	5.2	4.9	4.6	4.4	4.2	4	3.8	3.6	3.5
15	7.8	7.4	6.9	6.6	6.2	6	5.7	5.4	5.2
20	10.4	9.8	9.3	8.8	8.3	7.9	7.6	7.2	6.9
25	13	12.2	11.6	11	10.4	9.9	9.5	9.1	8.7
30	15.6	14.7	13.9	13.2	12.5	11.9	11.4	10.9	10.4

Inamrinone (Inocor)

Dose (mcg/kg/min) = CF × Rate (mL/hr).

Calculation Factors (CF) by Patient Weight (80-120 kg)

kg	80	85	90	95	100	105	110	115	120
CF	0.521	0.490	0.463	0.439	0.417	0.397	0.378	0.362	0.347

Infliximab (Remicade)

USES

1. Infliximab is a chimeric IgG1 monoclonal antibody that binds to human tumor necrosis factor alpha (TNF-α).
2. In combination with methotrexate, it is indicated for the treatment of rheumatoid arthritis.
3. It is also indicated as treatment for moderate to severe active Crohn's disease and fistulizing Crohn's disease.

SOLUTION PREPARATION

1. Infliximab is a sterile, white, lyophilized powder for IV infusion. It is in a single-use 20-mL vial of 100 mg. Infliximab should be stored in the refrigerator at 2°-8° C (36°-46° F).
2. Reconstitute with 10 mL of sterile water for injection. Swirl the vial to dissolve the powder; do not shake. Let stand for 5 minutes. Dilute to 250 mL with 0.9% sodium chloride. Mix gently. Infuse over a minimum of 2 hours, with an in-line, sterile, nonpyrogenic, low-protein binding filter of less than 1.2 mcm pore. The infusion should be started within 3 hours of preparation.

DOSE

1. *Rheumatoid arthritis:* 3 mg/kg as IV infusion, with next doses at 2 and 6 weeks, repeating dose every 8 weeks. Given with methotrexate.
2. *Active Crohn's disease:* 5 mg/kg as a single IV infusion.
3. *Fistulizing Crohn's disease:* 5 mg/kg but should be repeated again at 2 and 6 weeks.

CONTRAINDICATIONS

1. Moderate to severe congestive heart failure (CHF).
2. Known hypersensitivity to murine proteins or other components of the medication.

WARNINGS

1. Infection is the most common complication encountered during therapy with infliximab.
   a. Caution in patients on immunosuppressive therapy.

b. Caution in patients with a clinically important, active infection or history of recurrent infection.
c. Discontinue if patient develops a serious infection.
d. Caution in patients from regions where histoplasmosis is endemic; weigh benefits versus risks.
2. Discontinue use if patient develops a lupus-like syndrome.

ADVERSE REACTIONS

1. The most common adverse reactions are infusion related (i.e., dyspnea, urticaria, hypotension, flushing, headache).
2. Other side effects can affect the respiratory and GI systems.

INCOMPATIBILITY

No compatibility studies have been done with infliximab. Therefore it is suggested not to infuse infliximab concomitantly in the same IV line as other agents.

NURSING CONSIDERATIONS

1. Monitor patients for signs and symptoms of infection while they are on infliximab.
2. Inspect the solution for foreign particles or discoloration before infusion. The solution should be clear to yellow colored, opalescent, with few translucent particles.

Infliximab (Remicade)

Infliximab (Remicade) Dosing Chart
(Due to the high cost, doses are usually rounded to the nearest whole vial size to avoid waste)

Rheumatoid arthritis
(Final concentration: 3 mg/kg dose, 0.4-4 mg/mL)

Patient weight	Dose (mg) (per NS 250 mL)
≤33 kg	100 mg
34-67 kg	200 mg
68-100 kg	300 mg
101-133 kg	400 mg

Crohn's disease
(Final concentration: 5 mg/kg dose, 0.4-4 mg/mL)

Patient weight	Dose (mg) (per NS 250 mL)
21-40 kg	200 mg
41-60 kg	300 mg
61-80 kg	400 mg
81-100 kg	500 mg
101-120 kg	600 mg

Infliximab (Remicade) Initial Infusion Rates for Each 250-ml Bag*

Time	Rate
Start-15 mins	10 mL/hr
15-30 mins	20 mL/hr
30-45 mins	40 mL/hr
45-60 mins	80 mL/hr
60-90 mins	150 mL/hr
90-120 mins	250 mL/hr

*Must be infused over at least 2 hours.

Insulin Drip

USES
For diabetic ketoacidosis and/or treatment of elevated blood glucose.

SOLUTION PREPARATION
An insulin drip is prepared by adding 100 units (1 mL) of regular human insulin to 250 mL of 0.9% NaCl.
Final concentration: 100 units/250 mL (2 units/5 mL).

DOSE
Initial infusion is started at 5-10 units/hr and increased hourly as needed to control elevated blood sugar.

WARNINGS
Monitor blood sugar as ordered; hypoglycemia is possible if sugars are controlled too rapidly.

ADVERSE REACTIONS
Hypoglycemia

INCOMPATIBILITY
Aminophylline
Bretylium
Chlorothiazide
Cytarabine
Dobutamine
Dopamine
Labetalol
Levofloxacin
Lidocaine
Methylprednisolone
Nafcillin
Norepinephrine
Octreotide
Pentobarbital
Phenytoin
Ranitidine
Secobarbital
Sodium bicarbonate
Thiopental

COMPATIBILITY
Amiodarone
Ampicillin
Ampicillin/sulbactam
Aztreonam
Bretylium
Cefazolin
Cefotetan
Cimetidine
Clarithromycin
Diltiazem
Dobutamine
Esmolol
Famotidine
Gentamicin

Heparin
Imipenem/cilastatin
Indomethacin
Lidocaine
Magnesium sulfate
Meperidine
Meropenem
Midazolam
Milrinone
Morphine
Nitroglycerin

Nitroprusside
Oxytocin
Pentobarbital
Potassium chloride
Propofol
Ritodrine
Sodium bicarbonate
Tacrolimus
Terbutaline
Ticarcillin/clavulanate
Verapamil

NURSING CONSIDERATIONS

1. Consult the Insulin Drip Rate Calculation Chart to determine the drip rate.
2. Insulin should be administered via an IV pump to ensure controlled infusion.
3. Closely monitor and document changes in blood sugar.

Insulin Drip

Insulin Drip Rate Calculation Chart
Insulin 100 units in 250 mL (Concentration: 2 units/5 mL)

Dose	Infusion rate
10 units/hr	25 mL/hr
15 units/hr	38 mL/hr
20 units/hr	50 mL/hr
25 units/hr	63 mL/hr
30 units/hr	75 mL/hr

Isoproterenol (Isuprel)

USES

1. Hemodynamically important bradycardia unresponsive to atropine.
2. Temporary control of atropine refractory heart block prior to pacemaker insertion.
3. Treatment of carotid sinus hypersensitivity, Stokes-Adams disease, or ventricular arrhythmias due to AV block.
4. May be useful in shock characterized by low cardiac output and intense vasoconstriction, which persists after adequate fluid replacement.
5. Control of bronchial spasm occurring during anesthesia.

SOLUTION PREPARATION

An isoproterenol infusion is prepared by adding 1 mg (1 ampule, 5 mL) isoproterenol to 250 mL D5W.
Final concentration: 4 mcg/mL.

DOSE

1. *Bradycardia:* An Isuprel infusion is usually initiated in adults at 5 mcg/min. Subsequent dosage is adjusted according to patient response and generally ranges from 2-20 mcg/min. (A small bolus dose of 0.02-0.06 mg may be given prior to the infusion.)
2. *Shock:* For treatment in shock, infusion rates of 0.5-5 mcg/min have been recommended.

WARNINGS

1. Do not use the Isuprel solution if a color precipitate is present.
2. Isoproterenol is contraindicated in patients with preexisting arrhythmias (especially tachycardia), other than those that may be responsive to treatment with isoproterenol. Isoproterenol is contraindicated in patients with tachycardia caused by digoxin intoxication.
3. Blood volume depletion should be corrected before isoproterenol is administered to patients in shock.
4. Administer caution to geriatric patients, diabetics, patients with renal or cardiovascular disease, hyperthyroidism, and/or those with a history of sensitivity to sympathomimetic amines.

5. If HR exceeds 110 beats/min or premature ventricular contractions or changes in the ECG develop, consider slowing infusion or discontinuing temporarily.
6. Use with caution, if at all, in patients receiving cyclopropane or halogenated hydrocarbon general anesthetic.
7. May increase myocardial oxygen requirement; therefore avoid in patients with myocardial infarction (MI).
8. Use with caution when hypokalemia is present.

ADVERSE REACTIONS

1. *Cardiovascular:* Tachycardia, palpitations, ventricular arrhythmias, precordial pain.
2. Vasodilation with a drop in BP.
3. *CNS:* Headache, nervousness, anxiety, mild tremor.

INCOMPATIBILITY

Alkaline solutions
Aminophylline
Furosemide
Lidocaine
Sodium bicarbonate

COMPATIBILITY

Amiodarone
Atracurium
Bretylium
Calcium chloride
Cimetidine
Cisatracurium
Dobutamine
Dopamine
Famotidine
Floxacillin
Heparin
Hydrocortisone
Inamrinone
Levofloxacin
Magnesium sulfate
Milrinone
Multivitamins
Pancuronium
Potassium chloride
Propofol
Ranitidine
Remifentanil
Sodium succinate
Succinylcholine
Tacrolimus
Vecuronium
Verapamil
Vitamin B complex
  with C

Isoproterenol (Isuprel)

Isoproterenol (Isuprel)

NURSING CONSIDERATIONS

1. Consult the Isuprel Drip Rate Calculation Chart to determine the drip rate.
2. Except in cardiac arrest situations, isoproterenol should be administered via an IV pump to ensure controlled infusion.
3. The patient's ECG and HR should be continuously monitored while isoproterenol is being titrated. The patient's BP should be monitored at 10-minute intervals when the dose of isoproterenol is being incrementally increased. After desired results are obtained, monitor BP readings at least hourly and document.
4. Closely monitor and document changes in rate, ECG, BP, urine output, CVP, and cardiac output. Monitor patients in shock for urine output and arterial blood gases.

Isoproterenol (Isuprel) Drip Rate Calculation Chart
Isoproterenol 1 mg in 250 mL (Concentration: 4 mcg/mL)

Dose	Infusion rate
2 mcg/min	30 mL/hr
3 mcg/min	45 mL/hr
4 mcg/min	60 mL/hr
5 mcg/min	75 mL/hr
6 mcg/min	90 mL/hr
7 mcg/min	105 mL/hr
8 mcg/min	120 mL/hr
9 mcg/min	135 mL/hr
10 mcg/min	150 mL/hr
11 mcg/min	165 mL/hr
12 mcg/min	180 mL/hr

Continued

Isoproterenol (Isuprel)

Isoproterenol (Isuprel) Drip Rate Calculation Chart—cont'd
Isoproterenol 1 mg in 250 mL (Concentration: 4 mcg/mL)

Dose	Infusion rate
13 mcg/min	195 mL/hr
14 mcg/min	210 mL/hr
15 mcg/min	225 mL/hr
16 mcg/min	240 mL/hr
17 mcg/min	255 mL/hr
18 mcg/min	270 mL/hr
19 mcg/min	285 mL/hr
20 mcg/min	300 mL/hr

Labetalol (Trandate)

USES
Treatment of elevated BP.

SOLUTION PREPARATION
To prepare a labetalol infusion, add 200 mg (40 mL) Trandate to 160 mL NS (total volume equals 200 mL). Final concentration: 1 mg/mL. Stable for 24 hours; also stable in D5W or LR.

DOSE
1. An initial dose of 20 mg (4 mL) Trandate IV, slow injection. Available as 5 mg/mL, in 20-mL and 40-mL multidose vials.
2. Additional 40 mg (8 mL) or 80 mg (16 mL) can be given at 10-minute intervals until the desired supine BP is achieved or a total of 300 mg/24 hr has been given.
3. For IV infusions, infuse up to 2 mg/min or 120 mL/hr to obtain desired BP control. See Labetalol Drip Rate Calculation Chart.

WARNINGS
1. Have patient in supine position and closely observe for postural hypotension, which may occur for up to 3 hours after IV doses.
2. Maximum effect occurs within 5 minutes of each injection.
3. Use with caution in patients with hyperreactive airways, congestive heart failure (CHF), diabetes, and hepatic dysfunction.
4. Contraindicated in patients with cardiogenic shock, uncompensated CHF, bradycardia, pulmonary edema, and heart block.
5. Reduce dose in presence of liver failure.

ADVERSE REACTIONS

1. Hypotension (postural and supine).
2. Breathing difficulty, CHF, irregular heartbeat, bradycardia, dizziness.

INCOMPATIBILITY

Amphotericin B
Ceftriaxone
Furosemide
Heparin
Insulin
Nafcillin
Sodium bicarbonate
Thiopental
Warfarin

COMPATIBILITY

Amikacin
Aminophylline
Amiodarone
Ampicillin
Butorphanol
Calcium gluconate
Cefazolin
Ceftazidime
Cimetidine
Clindamycin
Chloramphenicol
Diltiazem
Dobutamine
Dopamine
Enalaprilat
Epinephrine
Erythromycin
Esmolol
Famotidine
Fentanyl
Gatifloxacin
Gentamicin
Heparin
Hydromorphone
Lidocaine
Linezolid
Lorazepam
Magnesium sulfate
Meperidine
Metronidazole
Midazolam
Milrinone
Morphine
Nicardipine
Nitroglycerin
Nitroprusside
Norepinephrine
Oxacillin
Penicillin G
Piperacillin
Potassium chloride
Propofol
Ranitidine
Tobramycin
Trimethoprim/sulfa
Vancomycin
Vecuronium

Labetalol (Trandate)

NURSING CONSIDERATIONS

1. Consult the Labetalol Drip Rate Calculation Chart to determine the drip rate.
2. Except in cardiac arrest situations, labetalol should be administered via an IV pump to ensure controlled infusion.
3. The patient's BP should be obtained upon labetalol administration and then at 5- and 10-minute intervals after each dose change; then every 30 minutes while on the infusion until stable. When BP has stabilized, monitor at least hourly and document.
4. Closely monitor and document changes in the ECG and HR.

Labetalol (Trandate) Drip Rate Calculation Chart
Trandate 200 mg/200 mL (Concentration: 1 mg/mL)

Dose	Infusion rate
0.5 mg/min	30 mL/hr
1 mg/min	60 mL/hr
1.5 mg/min	90 mL/hr
2 mg/min	120 mL/hr

Lepirudin (Refludan)

USES

Anticoagulation in patients with heparin-induced thrombocytopenia (HIT) and associated thromboembolic disorders to prevent further embolic complications.

SOLUTION PREPARATION

Lepirudin is mixed as 100 mg (2 mL) lepirudin in 250 mL NS. The final concentration is 0.4 mg/mL. The initial bolus dose is obtained from the 50-mg vial, reconstitute with 1 mL of sterile water or NS. The total contents of the vial should be withdrawn into a 10-mL syringe and further diluted to a total volume of 10 mL (equivalent to 5 mg/mL). See the dosing chart for the appropriate weight and volume to give IV push over 15-20 seconds.

DOSE

1. *IV bolus:* 0.4 mg/kg body weight up to 110 kg.
2. *IV infusion:* 0.15 mg/kg (up to 110 kg) for 2-10 days as indicated.

WARNINGS

1. Hemorrhage can occur at virtually any site in patients receiving lepirudin. An unexplained fall in hematocrit, fall in BP, or any other unexplained symptom should lead to serious consideration of a hemorrhagic event.
2. Use lepirudin with extreme caution in patients with disease states in which there is increased danger of hemorrhage (e.g., dissecting aneurysm, increased capillary permeability, severe hypertension, spinal anesthesia, GI ulceration, diverticulitis or ulcerative colitis, and liver disease with impaired hemostasis).

ADVERSE REACTIONS

1. *Incidence >10%:* Bleeding from puncture sites, wounds; anemia or drop in hemoglobin or hematoma formation.
2. *Incidence 1%-10%:* Fever, allergic skin reactions, GI or rectal bleeding, hematuria, vaginal bleeding, abnormal liver function tests, epistaxis, and hemothorax.

INCOMPATIBILITY

None reported.

COMPATIBILITY

None known.

NURSING CONSIDERATIONS

1. Consult the Lepirudin Drip Rate Calculation Chart to determine drip rate.
2. Lepirudin should be administered via an IV pump to ensure controlled infusion.
3. Monitor patients for signs/symptoms of hemorrhage; contact physician if symptoms occur.
4. Avoid IM injections.
5. Monitor PTT 4 hours after dose is initiated, then every morning. Therapeutic range is generally 1.5-2.5 times normal control, or about 55-80 seconds.
6. Reduce the infusion rate for patients with reduced renal function according to the following chart.

Creatinine clearance	Serum creatinine	Percent of standard drip	Dose (mg/kg/hr)
45-60	1.6-2	50%	0.075
30-44	2.1-3	30%	0.045
15-29	3.1-6	15%	0.023
Below 15	Above 6	Avoid use	Avoid use

Lepirudin (Refludan)

Lepirudin (Refludan)

Lepirudin (Refludan) Bolus Dosing Chart

To obtain the bolus dose, prepare a solution of 5 mg/mL final concentration as follows:
1. Reconstitute one 50-mg vial with 1 mL NS or sterile water.
2. Transfer the contents of the vial to a 10-mL syringe, and dilute to a total volume of 10 mL.
3. The final bolus dose based on patient's weight is withdrawn and given over 15-20 seconds.

Patient weight	Bolus volume 0.4 mg/kg (Normal renal function)	Bolus volume 0.2 mg/kg (Renal insufficiency: Cr >1.5 or CrCl <60)
50 kg	4 mL	2 mL
60 kg	4.8 mL	2.4 mL
70 kg	5.6 mL	2.8 mL
80 kg	6.4 mL	3.2 mL
90 kg	7.2 mL	3.6 mL
100 kg	8 mL	4 mL
≥110 kg	8.8 mL	4.4 mL

Lepirudin (Refludan) Drip Rate Calculation Chart for Normal Renal Function
Refludan 100 mg/250 mL (Concentration: 0.4 mg/mL)
Infusion rate 0.15 mg/kg/hr

Patient weight	Infusion rate
50 kg	19 mL/hr
60 kg	23 mL/hr
70 kg	26 mL/hr
80 kg	30 mL/hr
90 kg	34 mL/hr
100 kg	38 mL/hr
≥110 kg	41 mL/hr

Lidocaine (Xylocaine)

USES

1. Treatment of ventricular arrhythmias including significant premature ventricular contractions, ventricular tachycardia, and ventricular fibrillation.
2. Suppression of ventricular ectopy and ventricular arrhythmias associated with myocardial infarction (MI).

SOLUTION PREPARATION

Lidocaine is available in a premixed solution of 2 g/500 mL.

DOSE

1. Initial bolus of 1 mg/kg or 50-100 mg IVP at rate of approximately 25-50 mg/min. May repeat ½ of original dose in 5-10 minutes if needed. Not to exceed 300 mg in 1 hour.
2. Lidocaine bolus may be given via endotracheal tube.
3. Infusion of 1-4 mg/min after IV bolus.
4. Potassium arrhythmias appear during a constant infusion of lidocaine; a small bolus dose and an increase in the infusion rate may be given simultaneously.

WARNINGS

1. Use with caution in patients with liver disease, congestive heart failure (CHF), marked hypoxia, severe respiratory depression, hypovolemia, or shock.
2. Use with caution in patients with sinus bradycardia or incomplete heart block.
3. May increase ventricular rate in patients with atrial fibrillation.
4. Concurrent administration of lidocaine with cimetidine or propranolol may result in increased serum concentrations of lidocaine with resultant toxicity.
5. For infusions lasting >24 hours, a dosage reduction may be necessary to avoid drug accumulation and potential toxicity.

6. Lidocaine is contraindicated in patients with hypersensitivity to the amide-type local anesthetics. No cross sensitivity is seen with procaine (Novocain), procainamide, or quinidine.
7. Lidocaine is contraindicated in patients with severe sinoatrial (SA), AV, or intraventricular heart block in absence of artificial pacemaker.
8. Lidocaine is contraindicated in patients with Adam-Stokes or Wolff-Parkinson-White syndromes.

ADVERSE REACTIONS

1. *Cardiovascular:* Effects including hypotension, arrhythmias, heart block, cardiovascular collapse, and bradycardia.
2. *CNS:* Reactions as manifested by confusion, agitation, nausea, vomiting, convulsions, coma, and death.
3. Severe adverse reactions are often preceded by somnolence and paresthesia.

INCOMPATIBILITY

Amphotericin B
Ampicillin
Cefazolin
Ceftriaxone
Dacarbazine
Epinephrine
Isoproterenol
Methohexital
Norepinephrine
Phenytoin
Sodium bicarbonate

COMPATIBILITY

Alteplase
Aminophylline
Amiodarone
Atracurium
Bretylium
Bupivacaine
Calcium chloride
Calcium gluconate
Cefazolin
Chloramphenicol
Chlorothiazide
Cimetidine
Ciprofloxacin
Cisatracurium
Clarithromycin
Clonidine
Dexamethasone
Digoxin
Diltiazem
Diphenhydramine
Dobutamine
Dopamine

Lidocaine (Xylocaine)

Enalaprilat
Ephedrine
Erythromycin
Etomidate
Famotidine
Fentanyl
Floxacillin
Flumazenil
Furosemide
Gatifloxacin
Glycopyrrolate
Haloperidol
Heparin
Hydrocortisone
Hydroxyzine
Inamrinone
Insulin
Ketamine
Labetalol

Levofloxacin
Linezolid
Meperidine
Mephentermine
Metoclopramide
Milrinone
Morphine
Nafcillin
Nitroglycerin
Nitroprusside
Penicillin G
Pentobarbital
Phenylephrine
Potassium chloride
Procainamide
Promazine
Propafenone
Propofol
Ranitidine

Sodium bicarbonate
Sodium phosphate
Streptokinase
Tetracaine

Theophylline
Tirofiban
Verapamil

NURSING CONSIDERATIONS

1. Consult the Lidocaine Drip Rate Calculation Chart to determine the drip rate.
2. Except in cardiac arrest situations, lidocaine should be administered via an IV pump to ensure controlled infusion.
3. Monitor the ECG constantly for prolongation at the PR interval or QRS complex and/or appearance of arrhythmias. Depending on the severity of the reaction, decrease or discontinue lidocaine immediately. Document changes in HR and BP. Observe patient carefully and document signs or symptoms of adverse CNS effects.

Lidocaine (Xylocaine) Drip Rate Calculation Chart
Lidocaine 2 g in 500 mL (Concentration: 4 mg/mL)

Dose	Infusion rate
1 mg/min	15 mL/hr
2 mg/min	30 mL/hr
3 mg/min	45 mL/hr
4 mg/min	60 mL/hr

Lorazepam (Ativan)

USES
To provide general sedation and relief of anxiety, especially as a preanesthetic, or in mechanical ventilation.

SOLUTION PREPARATION
To prepare Ativan infusion, add 40 mg (10 mL of 4-mg/mL vial) Ativan to 500 mL D5W using a glass bottle only (not a PVC bag). **Final concentration:** 0.08 mg/mL.
NOTE: Solubility is 3 times greater in D5W than in NS. Maximum concentration for fluid-restricted patients is 80 mg in 500 mL D5W (0.16 mg/mL) in a glass bottle only.
Alternatively, Ativan may be infused undiluted directly from the 10-ml bottles using microbore tubing and a PCA pump set on continuous mode. This may avoid the problem of crystallization that can sometimes occur with diluted solutions.

DOSE
Continuous infusion:
1. Start 1 mg/hr, titrate up to 5 mg/hr.
2. Titrate dose to effect.
3. Increase dose as needed to achieve desired degree of sedation.

WARNINGS
1. Use with caution in patients with renal or hepatic impairment, organic brain syndrome (OBS), myasthenia gravis, or Parkinson's disease.
2. Filter (0.22 mcm) all solutions to avoid possible administration of any precipitated material.

ADVERSE REACTIONS
1. *Incidence 10%:* Hypotension, laryngospasm, rash, tachycardia, confusion, apnea, and decreased respiration.
2. *Incidence 1%-10%:* Bradycardia.

INCOMPATIBILITY

Aldesleukin
Atracurium
Aztreonam
Buprenorphine
Dexamethasone
Floxacillin
Foscarnet

Idarubicin
Imipenem/cilastatin
Ranitidine
Sargramostim
Sufentanil
Thiopental
Zofran

COMPATIBILITY

Acyclovir
Albumin
Allopurinol
Amifostine
Amikacin
Amphotericin B
Atracurium
Bumetanide
Cefepime
Cefotaxime
Cimetidine
Ciprofloxacin

Cisatracurium
Cisplatin
Cladribine
Clonidine
Cyclophosphamide
Cytarabine
Dexamethasone
Diltiazem
Dobutamine
Docetaxel
Dopamine
Doxorubicin

Epinephrine
Erythromycin
Etomidate
Etoposide
Famotidine
Fentanyl
Filgrastim
Fluconazole
Fludarabine
Fosphenytoin
Furosemide
Gatifloxacin
Gemcitabine
Gentamicin
Granisetron
Haloperidol
Heparin
Hydrocortisone
Hydromorphone
Labetalol
Levofloxacin
Linezolid

Methotrexate
Metronidazole
Midazolam
Milrinone
Morphine
Nicardipine
Nitroglycerin
Norepinephrine
Paclitaxel
Pancuronium
Piperacillin
Piperacillin/tazobactam
Potassium chloride
Propofol
Ranitidine
Tacrolimus
Teniposide
Thiotepa
Vancomycin
Vecuronium
Vinorelbine
Zidovudine

Lorazepam (Ativan)

Lorazepam (Ativan)

NURSING CONSIDERATIONS

1. Use with caution in the elderly, smaller doses may be needed to prevent side-effects (hypoventilation).
2. Avoid administering via small veins to prevent extravasation. Arterial administration should also be avoided because it may result in arteriospasm, gangrene, and amputation.
3. Patients may require assistance for up to 8 hours after the infusion is stopped.

Lorazepam (Ativan) Drip Rate Calculation Chart
Ativan 40 mg in 500 mL (Concentration: 0.08 mg/mL)

Dose	Infusion rate
1 mg/hr	12 mL/hr
2 mg/hr	25 mL/hr
3 mg/hr	37 mL/hr
4 mg/hr	50 mL/hr
5 mg/hr	63 mL/hr

Midazolam (Versed)

USES
To provide general sedation and relaxation during mechanical ventilation to prevent ventilator resistance and/or decreased energy expenditure states.

SOLUTION PREPARATION
To prepare Versed infusion, add 125 mg (25 mL of 5 mg/mL) Versed to 100 mL NS. **Final concentration: 1.0 mg/mL.**

DOSE
Continuous infusion:
1. Start 1 mg/hr; titrate up to 10 mg/hr.
2. Titrate dose to effect.
3. Increase dose as needed to achieve desired degree of sedation.

WARNINGS
Use with caution in patients with congestive heart failure (CHF), renal and hepatic dysfunction, and with concomitant narcotics.

ADVERSE REACTIONS
Hiccups (10%), bradycardia, hypotension, drowsiness, respiratory depression, amnesia.

INCOMPATIBILITY
Albumin
Amphotericin B
Ampicillin
Bumetanide
Butorphanol
Ceftazidime
Cefuroxime
Clonidine
Dexamethasone
Dimenhydrinate
Dobutamine
Floxacillin
Foscarnet
Fosphenytoin
Furosemide
Hydrocortisone
Imipenem/cilastatin
Methotrexate
Nafcillin
Phenobarbital
Prochlorperazine
Propofol
Ranitidine
Sodium bicarbonate
Thiopental
Trimethoprim/sulfa

COMPATIBILITY

Amiodarone
Amikacin
Atracurium
Atropine
Buprenorphine
Butorphanol
Calcium gluconate
Cefazolin
Cefotaxime
Chlorpromazine
Cimetidine
Ciprofloxacin
Cisatracurium
Clindamycin
Digoxin
Diltiazem
Diphenhydramine
Dopamine

Droperidol
Epinephrine
Erythromycin
Esmolol
Famotidine
Fentanyl
Gatifloxacin
Gentamicin
Haloperidol
Heparin
Hydromorphone
Hydroxyzine
Insulin
Labetalol
Linezolid
Lorazepam
Meperidine
Methylprednisolone

Metoclopramide
Metronidazole
Milrinone
Morphine
Nicardipine
Nitroglycerin
Nitroprusside
Ondansetron
Pancuronium

Piperacillin
Potassium chloride
Promethazine
Ranitidine
Theophylline
Tobramycin
Vancomycin
Vecuronium

NURSING CONSIDERATIONS

1. Flumazenil (Romazicon) is effective in reversing the effects of midazolam.
2. Elderly patients may require lower doses and be more sensitive to the respiratory depressant effects of midazolam.
3. Continuous monitoring of cardiac (BP, HR) and respiratory function (pulse oximetry) is usually required.

Midazolam (Versed)

Midazolam (Versed)

Midazolam (Versed) Drip Rate Calculation Chart
Versed 125 mg in 125 mL (Concentration: 1 mg/mL)

Dose	Infusion rate
1 mg/hr	1 mL/hr
3 mg/hr	3 mL/hr
5 mg/hr	5 mL/hr
7 mg/hr	7 mL/hr
10 mg/hr	10 mL/hr

Milrinone (Primacor)

USES

For short-term treatment of severe congestive heart failure (CHF) in patients who have not responded adequately to digitalis, diuretics, and/or vasodilators. Milrinone has vasodilatory and positive inotropic effects.

SOLUTION PREPARATION

A milrinone drip is prepared by adding 20 mg (1 vial) milrinone to 80 mL D5W or 0.9% NaCl. **Final concentration:** 20 mg/100 mL (200 mcg/mL). Premixed bag 20 mg/100 mL D5W is also available.

DOSE

1. Initial bolus of 50 mcg/kg given slowly over 10 minutes.
2. Maintenance infusion between 0.375 and 0.75 mcg/kg/min.
3. Total daily dose including boluses and cumulative infused dose should not exceed 1.13 mg/kg.

WARNINGS

1. May aggravate symptoms of idiopathic hypertrophic subsonic stenosis.
2. Supraventricular and ventricular arrhythmias have been observed. Some patients experienced increased ventricular ectopy, including nonsustained ventricular tachycardia.
3. Milrinone produces shortening of AV node conduction time, indicating a potential for an increased ventricular response rate in patients with atrial fibrillation/flutter that is not controlled with digitalis therapy.
4. If prior vigorous diuretic therapy is suspected to have caused significant decreases in cardiac filling pressure, milrinone should be cautiously administered with monitoring of BP, HR, and clinical symptomatology.
5. Milrinone not recommended in the acute phase of post-myocardial infarction (MI).
6. Dosage reduction is required in patents with renal impairment.

7. Milrinone-induced improvement in cardiac output with resultant diuresis may necessitate a reduction in the dose of diuretics.
8. Potassium loss resulting from excessive diuresis may predispose digitalized patients to arrhythmias. Hypokalemia should be corrected in advance of or during use of milrinone.

ADVERSE REACTIONS

1. Cardiac arrhythmias.
2. Hypotension.
3. Angina/chest pain.
4. Mild to moderate headache.
5. Thrombocytopenia (occurs rarely).

INCOMPATIBILITY

Bumetanide   Procainamide
Furosemide

COMPATIBILITY

Atracurium
Atropine
Calcium chloride
Calcium gluconate
Cimetidine
Digoxin
Diltiazem
Dobutamine
Dopamine
Epinephrine
Fentanyl
Heparin
Hydromorphone
Insulin
Isoproterenol
Labetalol
Lidocaine
Lorazepam
Magnesium sulfate
Midazolam
Morphine
Nicardipine
Nitroglycerin
Nitroprusside
Norepinephrine
Pancuronium
Potassium chloride
Propofol
Propranolol
Quinidine gluconate
Ranitidine
Sodium bicarbonate
Theophylline
Thiopental
Torsemide
Vecuronium
Verapamil

Milrinone (Primacor)

NURSING CONSIDERATIONS

1. Depending on the patient's status, an accurate weight should be obtained before the administration of milrinone.
2. Consult the Milrinone Drip Rate Calculation Chart to determine the drip rate.
3. BP should be measured every 15 minutes until stable, then at least hourly as long as drip remains in use.
4. Closely monitor and document changes in CVP, HR, urine output, body weight, and clinical signs of CHF (e.g., orthopnea, dyspnea, and fatigue).

Milrinone (Primacor) Drip Rate Calculation Chart
Milrinone 20 mg in 100 mL (Concentration: 0.2 mg/mL)
Infusion Rates (mL/hr); Standard Premixed Drug Concentration 20 mg in 100 mL
(0.2 mg/mL)

Patient weight (kg)	Patient weight (lb)	0.375 (mcg/kg/min mL/hr)	0.5 (mcg/kg/min mL/hr)	0.75 (mcg/kg/min mL/hr)
40	88	4.5	6	9
45	99	5.1	6.8	10.1
50	110	5.6	7.5	11.3
55	121	6.2	8.2	12.4
60	132	6.8	9	13.5
65	143	7.3	9.8	14.6
70	154	7.9	10.5	15.8
75	165	8.4	11.2	16.9
80	176	9	12	18
85	187	9.6	12.7	19.1
90	198	10.1	13.5	20.3
95	209	10.7	14.2	21.4
100	220	11.3	15	22.5

Continued

Milrinone (Primacor)

Milrinone (Primacor) Drip Rate Calculation Chart—cont'd
Milrinone 20 mg in 100 mL (Concentration: 0.2 mg/mL)
Infusion Rates (mL/hr); Standard Premixed Drug Concentration 20 mg in 100 mL
(0.2 mg/mL)

Patient weight (kg)	Patient weight (lb)	0.375 (mcg/kg/min mL/hr)	0.5 (mcg/kg/min mL/hr)	0.75 (mcg/kg/min mL/hr)
105	231	11.8	15.7	23.6
110	242	12.4	16.5	24.8
115	253	12.9	17.2	25.9
120	264	13.5	18	27
125	275	14	18.7	28.1
130	286	14.6	19.5	29.2
135	297	15.2	20.2	30.4

Nesiritide (Natrecor)

USES

Intravenous treatment of patients with acutely decompensated congestive heart failure (CHF) who have dyspnea at rest or with minimal activity. Nesiritide reduces pulmonary capillary wedge pressure and improves dyspnea.

SOLUTION PREPARATION

1. Reconstitute 1.5 mg vial with 5 mL of diluent from 250-mL bag of desired IV fluid by gently rocking vial. Do not shake. *Solution should be colorless.*
2. Withdraw entire contents of vial and add to the 250-mL bag. Resulting solution yields a 6 mcg/mL concentration.
3. Invert IV bag to ensure mixing.
4. Use within 24 hours. May be stored at room temperature.

DOSE

1. Initial bolus dose of 2 mcg/kg followed by infusion of 0.01 mcg/kg/min. See dosing chart.

2. *Dosage adjustment:* If hypotension occurs, the infusion rate should be decreased or stopped and other measures to support BP should be started. Natrecor may be restarted at a 30% reduced dose once the patient has stabilized (a period of observation may be necessary prior to restarting Natrecor).
3. *To increase dose:* Administer a new bolus of 1 mcg/kg and increase the infusion rate by 0.005 mcg/kg/min.
4. *Maximum infusion rate is 0.03 mcg/kg/min.* Doses should usually only be given for 48 hours.

WARNINGS

1. Care should be taken when administering Natrecor with other medications known to cause hypotension.
2. *Never exceed the recommended dose.*

ADVERSE REACTIONS

1. Back pain.
2. Headache.
3. Hypotension (most common).
4. Nausea.
5. Ventricular tachycardia.

INCOMPATIBILITY

Bumetanide
Enalaprilat
Ethacrynate acid
Furosemide
Heparin*

Hydralazine
Injectable drugs with the
  preservative sodium
  metabisulfite
Insulin

*Do not administer via heparin-coated central catheter.

COMPATIBLE SOLUTIONS

Dextrose 5% in water
Normal saline

Dextrose 5% ½NS
Dextrose 5% ¼NS

NURSING CONSIDERATIONS

1. Obtain appropriate weight.
2. Avoid using in patients with cardiogenic shock, SBP <90 mm Hg, or low cardiac filling pressures.
3. Monitor blood pressure closely.
4. Do not exceed recommended doses.
5. If hypotension occurs, Natrecor should be stopped or rate of infusion decreased.
6. Hypotensive effects of Natrecor may last hours after infusion stopped.

Nesiritide (Natrecor)

Nesiritide (Natrecor)

Nesiritide (Natrecor) Weight-Adjusted Bolus Volume and Infusion Flow Rates
(2 mcg/kg Bolus Followed by a 0.01 mcg/kg/min Dose)
(Final Concentration: 6 mcg/mL)
(1.5 mg Nesiritide in 250 mL Diluent)

| Weight range | | | | |
lbs	kg	Bolus volume	Maintenance infusion rate	Maximum infusion rate
132	60	20 mL	6 mL/hr	18 mL/hr
154	70	23.3 mL	7 mL/hr	21 mL/hr
176	80	26.7 mL	8 mL/hr	24 mL/hr
198	90	30 mL	9 mL/hr	27 mL/hr
220	100	33.3 mL	10 mL/hr	30 mL/hr
242	110	36.7 mL	11 mL/hr	33 mL/hr

Nitroglycerin

USES

1. Treatment of angina in patients who have not responded to recommended doses of organic nitrates and/or beta-blockers.
2. Congestive heart failure (CHF) associated with acute myocardial infarction (AMI).
3. Control of BP in perioperative hypertension.
4. Production of controlled hypotension during surgical procedures.

SOLUTION PREPARATION

Premixed nitroglycerin solutions are available as a 25-mg/250-mL D5W solution (100 mcg/mL).

DOSE

The usual starting dose is 5 mcg/min. Increase infusion by 5 mcg/min every 3-5 minutes until desired response is obtained (e.g., predetermined hemodynamic state such as BP or PCWP, or pain relief). If no effect is obtained with 20 mcg/min, the infusion may be increased by 10 mcg/min increments. Once a partial BP response is obtained, increases in dosage increments should be reduced and the interval between dosage increases should be lengthened. The usual maximum dose is 200 mcg/min.

When discontinuing a drip, decrease dosage by 5 mcg/min increments and carefully monitor patient response.

WARNINGS

1. IV nitroglycerin is contraindicated in patients with hypotension or uncorrected hypovolemia.
2. IV nitroglycerin is contraindicated in patients with constrictive pericarditis and pericardial tamponade.
3. IV nitroglycerin is contraindicated in patients with severe anemia.
4. IV nitroglycerin is contraindicated in patients with previous idiosyncratic or hypersensitivity reaction.
5. Use with caution, if at all, in patients with increased intracranial pressure (e.g., head trauma, cerebral hemorrhage).

ADVERSE REACTIONS

1. Hypotension.
2. Headache, flushing, dizziness.
3. Nausea, vomiting.
4. Bradycardia.
5. Methemoglobinemia with very large doses (blue skin and mucous membranes, vomiting, shock, coma).

INCOMPATIBILITY

Do not mix nitroglycerin in the same bottle with any other drugs.

COMPATIBILITY (VIA Y SITE)

Amiodarone
Amphotericin B
Atracurium
Cisatracurium
Diltiazem
Dobutamine
Dopamine
Epinephrine
Esmolol
Famotidine
Fentanyl
Fluconazole
Furosemide
Gatifloxacin
Haloperidol
Heparin
Hydromorphone
Inamrinone
Insulin
Labetalol
Lidocaine
Linezolid
Lorazepam
Midazolam
Milrinone
Morphine
Nicardipine
Nitroprusside
Norepinephrine
Pancuronium
Propofol
Ranitidine
Streptokinase
Tacrolimus
Theophylline
Thiopental
Vecuronium
Warfarin

NURSING CONSIDERATIONS

1. Consult the Nitroglycerin Drip Rate Calculation Chart to determine the drip rate.
2. Except in cardiac arrest situations, nitroglycerin should be administered via an IV pump to ensure controlled infusion.

Nitroglycerin

3. The patient's BP should be monitored with each increase in dose while nitroglycerin is being incrementally increased. After the desired results are obtained, monitor BP at least hourly and document. Any disproportionate rise or fall in BP should be noted and reported immediately to the physician.
4. Closely monitor and document changes in HR, renal output, PCWP, cardiac output, and pain relief.

Nitroglycerin Drip Rate Calculation Chart
Nitroglycerin 25 mg in 250 mL (Concentration: 100 mcg/mL)

Dose	Infusion rate
5 mcg/min	3 mL/hr
10 mcg/min	6 mL/hr
15 mcg/min	9 mL/hr
20 mcg/min	12 mL/hr
30 mcg/min	18 mL/hr
40 mcg/min	24 mL/hr
50 mcg/min	30 mL/hr
60 mcg/min	36 mL/hr
70 mcg/min	42 mL/hr
80 mcg/min	48 mL/hr
90 mcg/min	54 mL/hr
100 mcg/min	60 mL/hr
110 mcg/min	66 mL/hr
120 mcg/min	72 mL/hr
130 mcg/min	78 mL/hr
140 mcg/min	84 mL/hr
150 mcg/min	90 mL/hr

Nitroprusside (Nipride)

USES

1. Immediate treatment of hypertensive crisis.
2. To produce controlled hypotension during surgery to minimize blood loss.
3. May be used for patients with refractory heart failure and/or acute myocardial infarction (AMI).
4. May be useful for patients with severe mitral regurgitation.

SOLUTION PREPARATION

Nitroprusside 50-mg vial is reconstituted with 2-3 mL D5W (no other diluent should be used) and added to 500 mL D5W. **Final concentration:** 50 mg/500 mL (100 mcg/mL). May also mix 100 mg in 250 mL D5W for final concentration of 400 mcg/mL (0.4 mg/mL).

Freshly prepared solutions have a faint brownish tint. Nitroprusside decomposes on exposure to light. It will change from a light brown to a dark brown, orange, or blue. Shield from light; when the solution is adequately protected from light, the reconstituted solution is stable for 24 hours. Discard the solution if it turns blue-green or dark brown.

DOSE

Effective infusion rates range from 0.5-8.0 mcg/kg/min. The dose may be titrated up slowly by 0.5-mcg/kg/min increments every 5 minutes until the desired pressure is achieved. Dosages should not exceed 10 mcg/kg/min. The effects of nitroprusside on BP are immediate.

WARNINGS

1. Nitroprusside is contraindicated in compensatory hypertension (e.g., arteriovenous shunt or coarctation of the aorta).
2. Thiocyanate and/or cyanide toxicity may occur when nitroprusside is administered at high doses or for a prolonged time and in patients with renal impairment or hepatic insufficiency.
3. Use with caution in patients with low vitamin B_{12} concentrations, hyperthyroidism, and hyponatremia.
4. Hypotensive effects are additive when used with ganglionic blocking agents, general anesthetics (halothane, enflurane), and with most other circulatory depressants.

ADVERSE REACTIONS

1. Profound hypotension.
2. Thiocyanate toxicity, which may cause a neurotoxic syndrome and symptoms of hypothyroidism.
3. Cyanide toxicity (metabolic acidosis is an early indicator).
4. Nausea, vomiting, diaphoresis, nasal stuffiness, muscular twitching, dizziness, and weakness; these are usually associated with rapid administration and can be reversed by decreasing the infusion rate.
5. Tolerance to the hypotensive effect.

INCOMPATIBILITY

No other drug should be added to the infusion fluid for simultaneous administration with nitroprusside.

COMPATIBILITY

Atracurium
Cimetidine
Diltiazem
Dobutamine
Dopamine
Enalaprilat
Esmolol
Famotidine
Heparin
Inamrinone
Indomethacin
Insulin
Labetalol
Lidocaine
Midazolam
Milrinone
Morphine
Nitroglycerin
Pancuronium
Propofol
Ranitidine
Tacrolimus
Theophylline
Verapamil
Vecuronium

NURSING CONSIDERATIONS

1. An accurate weight should be obtained before administration of nitroprusside.
2. Consult the Nitroprusside Drip Rate Calculation Chart to determine the drip rate.
3. Nitroprusside should be administered via an IV pump to ensure controlled infusion.
4. The patient's BP should be monitored by an arterial line or Swan-Ganz catheter (if this is not possible, a cuff BP should be taken) every time

Nitroprusside (Nipride)

Nitroprusside (Nipride)

the dose of nitroprusside is incrementally increased. After the desired results are obtained, monitor BP at least hourly and document. If nitroprusside is maintained at the same rate and the BP is stable for an entire shift, then the BP may be checked at 1-hour intervals. Any disproportionate rise or fall in BP should be noted and reported immediately to the physician.

5. Closely observe for signs and symptoms of toxicity, which include profound hypotension, increasing tolerance to the hypotensive effects of nitroprusside, metabolic acidosis, dyspnea, headache, vomiting, dizziness, ataxia, and loss of consciousness. If observed, notify the attending physician immediately and recommend discontinuation.

NOTE: The recommended medical treatment for overdosage includes amyl nitrite inhalation, 3% sodium nitrate IV solution, sodium thiosulfate solution, or a cyanide antidote kit.

Nitroprusside (Nipride) Drip Rate Calculation Chart—
Patient Weight 45-90 kg (99-199 lbs)
Regular Strength (Concentration: 0.1 mg/mL [50 mg/500 mL])

lbs kg	99 45	110 50	121 55	132 60	143 65	154 70	165 75	176 80	189 85	199 90
mL/hr	Dose = mcg/kg/min									
10	0.37	0.33	0.31	0.28	0.26	0.24	0.23	0.21	0.19	0.19
15	0.56	0.50	0.46	0.41	0.38	0.36	0.33	0.31	0.29	0.28
20	0.74	0.67	0.61	0.56	0.51	0.48	0.44	0.42	0.39	0.36
25	0.93	0.84	0.76	0.69	0.64	0.59	0.56	0.53	0.49	0.46
30	1.11	1	0.91	0.83	0.74	0.71	0.67	0.63	0.59	0.56
35	1.29	1.16	1.06	0.97	0.90	0.83	0.78	0.73	0.69	0.64
40	1.48	1.33	1.21	1.11	1.02	0.95	0.89	0.83	0.79	0.74
45	1.66	1.50	1.36	1.25	1.15	1.06	1	0.94	0.88	0.83
50	1.85	1.67	1.50	1.39	1.28	1.19	1.11	1.04	0.98	0.93
55	2.03	1.83	1.66	1.53	1.41	1.31	1.22	1.14	1.08	1.02

Continued

Nitroprusside (Nipride)

Nitroprusside (Nipride)

Nitroprusside (Nipride) Drip Rate Calculation Chart—Patient Weight 45-90 kg (99-199 lbs)—cont'd
Regular Strength (Concentration: 0.1 mg/mL [50 mg/500 mL])

lbs	99	110	121	132	143	154	165	176	189	199
kg	45	50	55	60	65	70	75	80	85	90
mL/hr	Dose = mcg/kg/min									
60	2.22	2	1.82	1.67	1.54	1.43	1.33	1.25	1.18	1.11
70	2.59	2.33	2.13	1.96	1.79	1.67	1.56	1.46	1.38	1.29
80	2.96	2.67	2.43	2.23	2.05	1.91	1.78	1.67	1.57	1.48
90	3.33	3	2.73	2.50	2.30	2.14	2	1.88	1.76	1.67

Dose (mcg/kg/min) = CF × Rate (mL/hr).

Calculation Factors (CF) by Patient Weight (45-90 kg) for Nipride 50 mg/500 mL

| kg | 45 | 50 | 55 | 60 | 65 | 70 | 75 | 80 | 85 | 90 |
| CF | 0.0370 | 0.0330 | 0.0300 | 0.0280 | 0.0260 | 0.0240 | 0.0220 | 0.0210 | 0.0200 | 0.0190 |

Nitroprusside (Nipride) Drip Rate Calculation Chart—
Patient Weight 95-150 kg (209-330 lbs)
Regular Strength (Concentration: 0.1 mg/mL [50 mg/500 mL])

lbs	209	220	231	242	253	264	273	286	297	330
kg	95	100	105	110	115	120	125	130	140	150
mL/hr	Dose = mcg/kg/min									
10	0.180	0.170	0.160	0.150	0.145	0.140	0.130	0.125	0.115	0.110
15	0.260	0.250	0.240	0.230	0.210	0.205	0.195	0.190	0.172	0.165
20	0.350	0.330	0.320	0.310	0.290	0.280	0.260	0.250	0.235	0.220
25	0.440	0.410	0.390	0.380	0.360	0.345	0.330	0.315	0.300	0.275
30	0.530	0.500	0.480	0.460	0.435	0.415	0.400	0.380	0.355	0.330
35	0.610	0.580	0.560	0.530	0.510	0.485	0.465	0.445	0.415	0.390
40	0.700	0.670	0.640	0.610	0.580	0.550	0.530	0.510	0.470	0.440
45	0.790	0.750	0.710	0.680	0.655	0.620	0.600	0.575	0.540	0.490
50	0.880	0.830	0.790	0.760	0.725	0.690	0.660	0.640	0.605	0.550
55	0.960	0.910	0.870	0.830	0.810	0.760	0.710	0.705	0.650	0.610

Continued

Nitroprusside (Nipride)

Nitroprusside (Nipride) Drip Rate Calculation Chart—Patient Weight 95-150 kg (209-330 lbs)—cont'd
Regular Strength (Concentration: 0.1 mg/mL [50 mg/500 mL])

lbs	209	220	231	242	253	264	273	286	297	330
kg	95	100	105	110	115	120	125	130	140	150
mL/hr	Dose = mcg/kg/min									
60	1.050	1	0.950	0.910	0.870	0.830	0.800	0.770	0.710	0.670
70	1.230	1.170	1.110	1.060	1.010	0.970	0.905	0.895	0.840	0.800
80	1.410	1.330	1.270	1.240	1.160	1.100	1.060	1.020	0.950	0.890
90	1.580	1.500	1.430	1.360	1.300	1.250	1.200	1.150	1.050	1

Dose (mcg/kg/min) = CF × Rate (mL/hr).

Calculation Factors (CF) by Patient Weight (95-150 kg) for Nipride 50 mg/500 mL

kg	95	100	105	110	115	120	125	130	140	150
CF	0.0180	0.0170	0.0160	0.0150	0.0145	0.0140	0.0133	0.0128	0.0118	0.0112

Nitroprusside (Nipride) Drip Rate Calculation Chart—
Patient Weight 45-110 kg (99-242 lbs)
Double Strength (Concentration: 0.2 mg/mL [50 mg/250 mL])

lbs	99	110	121	132	143	154	165	176	189	199	209	220	231	242
kg	45	50	55	60	65	70	75	80	85	90	95	100	105	110
mL/hr							Dose = mcg/kg/min							
10	0.74	0.66	0.69	0.56	0.52	0.48	0.46	0.42	0.38	0.38	0.36	0.34	0.32	0.30
15	1.22	1	0.92	0.82	0.76	0.72	0.66	0.62	0.58	0.56	0.52	0.50	0.48	0.46
20	1.48	1.34	1.22	1.12	1.01	0.93	0.88	0.84	0.78	0.72	0.70	0.66	0.64	0.62
25	1.86	1.68	1.52	1.38	1.28	1.18	1.12	1.06	0.98	0.92	0.88	0.82	0.78	0.76
30	2.22	2	1.82	1.66	1.48	1.42	1.34	1.26	1.18	1.12	1.06	1	0.96	0.92
35	2.58	2.32	2.12	1.94	1.80	1.76	1.56	1.42	1.38	1.28	1.22	1.16	1.12	1.06
40	2.96	2.66	2.42	2.22	2.04	1.90	1.78	1.63	1.58	1.48	4.40	1.34	1.28	1.22
45	3.32	3	2.72	2.50	2.30	2.12	2	1.88	1.76	1.66	1.58	1.50	1.42	1.36
50	3.70	3.34	3	2.78	2.56	2.38	2.22	2.08	1.96	1.86	1.76	1.66	1.58	1.52
55	4.06	3.66	3.32	3.06	2.82	2.62	2.44	2.38	2.16	2.04	1.92	1.82	1.74	1.66

Nitroprusside (Nipride)

Nitroprusside (Nipride)

Nitroprusside (Nipride) Drip Rate Calculation Chart—Patient Weight 45-110 kg (99-242 lbs)—cont'd
Double Strength (Concentration: 0.2 mg/mL [50 mg/250 mL])

lbs	99	110	121	132	143	154	165	176	189	199	209	220	231	242
kg	45	50	55	60	65	70	75	80	85	90	95	100	105	110
mL/hr						Dose = mcg/kg/min								
60	4.44	4	3.64	3.34	3.08	2.86	2.66	2.50	2.36	2.22	2.10	2	1.90	1.80
70	5.18	4.66	4.26	3.88	3.58	3.34	3.12	2.92	2.76	2.58	2.46	2.34	2.22	2.12
80	5.92	5.34	4.86	4.46	4.10	3.82	3.56	3.34	3.14	2.96	2.82	2.66	2.54	2.48
90	6.66	6	5.46	5	4.60	4.28	4	3.76	3.52	3.34	3.16	3	2.86	2.72

Dose (mcg/kg/min) = CF × Rate (mL/hr).

Calculation Factors (CF) by Patient Weight (45-75 kg) for Nipride 50 mg/250 mL

kg	45	50	55	60	65	70	75
CF	0.074	0.067	0.061	0.056	0.051	0.048	0.044

Calculation Factors (CF) by Patient Weight (80-110 kg) for Nipride 50 mg/250 mL

kg	80	85	90	95	100	105	110
CF	0.042	0.039	0.037	0.035	0.033	0.032	0.030

**Nitroprusside (Nipride) Drip Rate Calculation Chart—
Patient Weight 45-110 kg (99-242 lbs)**
Quadruple Strength (Concentration: 0.4 mg/mL [100 mg/250 mL])

lbs	99	110	121	132	143	154	165	176	189	199	209	220	231	242
kg	**45**	**50**	**55**	**60**	**65**	**70**	**75**	**80**	**85**	**90**	**95**	**100**	**105**	**110**
mL/hr						Dose = mcg/kg/min								
5	0.74	0.66	0.69	0.56	0.52	0.48	0.46	0.42	0.38	0.38	0.36	0.34	0.32	0.30
7.5	1.22	1	0.92	0.82	0.76	0.72	0.66	0.62	0.58	0.56	0.52	0.50	0.48	0.46
10	1.48	1.34	1.22	1.12	1.01	0.93	0.88	0.84	0.78	0.72	0.70	0.66	0.64	0.62
12.5	1.86	1.68	1.52	1.38	1.28	1.18	1.12	1.06	0.98	0.92	0.88	0.82	0.78	0.76
15	2.22	2	1.82	1.66	1.48	1.42	1.34	1.26	1.18	1.12	1.06	1	0.96	0.92
17.5	2.58	2.32	2.12	1.94	1.80	1.76	1.56	1.42	1.38	1.28	1.22	1.16	1.12	1.06
20	2.96	2.66	2.42	2.22	2.04	1.90	1.78	1.63	1.58	1.48	4.40	1.34	1.28	1.22
22.5	3.32	3	2.72	2.50	2.30	2.12	2	1.88	1.76	1.66	1.58	1.50	1.42	1.36
25	3.70	3.34	3	2.78	2.56	2.38	2.22	2.08	1.96	1.86	1.76	1.66	1.58	1.52
27.5	4.06	3.66	3.32	3.06	2.82	2.62	2.44	2.38	2.16	2.04	1.92	1.82	1.74	1.66

Continued

Nitroprusside (Nipride)

Nitroprusside (Nipride) Drip Rate Calculation Chart—
Patient Weight 45-110 kg (99-242 lbs)
Quadruple Strength (Concentration: 0.4 mg/mL [100 mg/250 mL])

lbs	99	110	121	132	143	154	165	176	189	199	209	220	231	242
kg	45	50	55	60	65	70	75	80	85	90	95	100	105	110
mL/hr						Dose = mcg/kg/min								
30	4.44	4	3.64	3.34	3.08	2.86	2.66	2.50	2.36	2.22	2.10	2	1.90	1.80
35	5.18	4.66	4.26	3.88	3.58	3.34	3.12	2.92	2.76	2.58	2.46	2.34	2.22	2.12
40	5.92	5.34	4.86	4.46	4.10	3.82	3.56	3.34	3.14	2.96	2.82	2.66	2.54	2.48
45	6.66	6	5.46	5	4.60	4.28	4	3.76	3.52	3.34	3.16	3	2.86	2.72

Dose (mcg/kg/min) = CF × Rate (mL/hr).

Calculation Factors (CF) by Patient Weight (45-75 kg) for Nipride 100 mg/250 mL

kg	45	50	55	60	65	70	75
CF	0.148	0.133	0.121	0.111	0.103	0.095	0.089

Calculation Factors (CF) by Patient Weight (80-110 kg) for Nipride 100 mg/250 mL

kg	80	85	90	95	100	105	110
CF	0.083	0.078	0.074	0.070	0.067	0.063	0.061

Norepinephrine (Levophed)

USES
1. Treatment of hypotension and shock via vasoconstriction and cardiac stimulation.
2. Adjunct in the therapy of cardiac arrest and profound hypotension.

SOLUTION PREPARATION
A norepinephrine drip is prepared by adding 4 mg (one 4-mg ampule) norepinephrine to 250 mL D5W. **Final concentration:** 4 mg/250 mL (16 mcg/mL), then add 5 mg (one 5-mg vial) of Regitine to each bag.

Levophed injection should not be used if it is brown in color or contains a precipitate.

DOSE
1. The usual initial adult dose is 8-12 mcg/min. The effect of the initial dose on BP is carefully observed and the infusion rate adjusted to establish and maintain the desired BP.
2. The average adult maintenance dose of norepinephrine is 2-4 mcg/min. Some patients require much higher doses. When discontinuing treatment, the infusion rate should be slowed gradually and abrupt withdrawal avoided.

WARNINGS
1. Norepinephrine increases myocardial oxygen consumption and the work of the heart.
2. Blood volume depletion should be corrected before norepinephrine therapy is instituted.
3. Hypoxia, hypercapnia, and acidosis should be corrected before norepinephrine therapy is begun.
4. Extravasation or peripheral ischemia can cause sloughing and necrosis of tissue in the surrounding area. **Antidote:** The site should be infiltrated with a 10-mL solution containing 5 mg phentolamine (Regitine); use a fine hypodermic needle.
5. In patients with severe hypotension after myocardial infarction (MI), thrombosis in the infused vein may be prevented by adding enough heparin to the infusion to supply 100-200 units/hr.

6. Levophed contains sodium metabisulfite and should be used with caution in patients with sensitivity to sulfiting agents.
7. Administer with caution in hypertensive or hyperthyroid patients.
8. Norepinephrine is contraindicated in patients with peripheral or mesenteric vascular thrombosis unless necessary as a lifesaving procedure.
9. Norepinephrine is contraindicated during anesthesia with cyclopropane or halogenated hydrocarbon anesthetics.
10. Use with caution and in low dose in patients taking tricyclic antidepressants, some antihistamines (e.g., diphenhydramine, tripelennamine, and dexchlorpheniramine), parenteral-ergot alkaloids, guanethidine, methyldopa, and MAO inhibitors (e.g., Marplan, Nardil, or Parnate).

ADVERSE REACTIONS

1. *Cardiovascular:* Arrhythmias (including bradycardia, bigeminal rhythms, ventricular tachycardia, ventricular fibrillation), precordial pain, severe hypertension.
2. *CNS:* Dizziness, anxiety, restlessness, headache, insomnia.
3. Severe peripheral and visceral vasoconstriction with decreased urine output, tissue hypoxia, and metabolic acidosis.
4. With overdosage one may see intense sweating, vomiting, retrosternal pain, hypertension, cerebral hemorrhage, and convulsions.

INCOMPATIBILITY

Aminophylline	Nafcillin
Amobarbital	Phenobarbital
Barbiturates	Phenytoin
Cephalothin	Sodium bicarbonate
Cephapirin	Streptomycin
Chlorothiazide	Thiopental
Insulin	Whole blood

Norepinephrine (Levophed)

Norepinephrine (Levophed)

COMPATIBILITY

Amikacin
Amiodarone
Calcium chloride
Calcium gluconate
Cimetidine
Cisatracurium
Corticotropin
Diltiazem
Dimenhydrinate
Dobutamine
Dopamine
Epinephrine
Esmolol
Famotidine
Fentanyl
Furosemide
Haloperidol
Heparin
Hydrocortisone
Hydromorphone
Inamrinone
Labetalol
Lorazepam
Magnesium sulfate
Meropenem
Methylprednisolone
Midazolam
Milrinone
Morphine
Multivitamins
Nicardipine
Nitroglycerin
Potassium chloride
Propofol
Ranitidine
Remifentanil
Succinylcholine
Vecuronium

NURSING CONSIDERATIONS

1. Consult the Norepinephrine Drip Rate Calculation Chart to determine the drip rate.
2. Except in cardiac arrest, norepinephrine should be administered via an IV pump to ensure controlled infusion.
3. The patent's BP should be monitored every 5 minutes from the time the norepinephrine infusion is started until the desired effect is achieved, then every 15 minutes while the drug is being infused.
4. Closely document changes in skin color or temperature in the extremities as a monitor for ischemia. Observe patients for extravasation. Closely document changes in HR, renal output, and ECG.

Norepinephrine (Levophed) Drip Rate Calculation Chart
Norepinephrine 4 mg in 250 mL (Concentration: 16 mcg/mL)

Dose	Infusion rate
2 mcg/min	8 mL/hr
3 mcg/min	11 mL/hr
4 mcg/min	15 mL/hr
5 mcg/min	19 mL/hr
6 mcg/min	22 mL/hr
7 mcg/min	26 mL/hr
8 mcg/min	30 mL/hr
9 mcg/min	34 mL/hr
10 mcg/min	38 mL/hr
11 mcg/min	41 mL/hr
12 mcg/min	45 mL/hr

Norepinephrine (Levophed)

**Norepinephrine (Levophed) Drip Rate Calculation Chart—
Patient Weight 35-70 kg (77-154 lbs)**
Concentration: 16 mcg/mL (1 ampule/250 mL)

lbs	77	88	99	110	121	132	143	154
kg	35	40	45	50	55	60	65	70
mL/hr				Dose = mcg/kg/min				
5	0.038	0.034	0.029	0.026	0.024	0.022	0.020	0.019
10	0.076	0.067	0.059	0.053	0.049	0.045	0.041	0.038
15	0.144	0.100	0.039	0.080	0.073	0.066	0.061	0.057
20	0.152	0.133	0.118	0.107	0.097	0.089	0.082	0.076
25	0.190	0.166	0.148	0.134	0.121	0.111	0.102	0.095
30	0.229	0.200	0.178	0.160	0.146	0.133	0.123	0.114
35	0.267	0.233	0.207	0.186	0.170	0.153	0.143	0.133
40	0.305	0.267	0.237	0.213	0.194	0.178	0.164	0.152
45	0.343	0.300	0.266	0.240	0.218	0.200	0.184	0.171
50	0.381	0.333	0.296	0.267	0.242	0.222	0.205	0.190
55	0.419	0.360	0.326	0.293	0.266	0.244	0.225	0.209
60	0.457	0.400	0.356	0.320	0.291	0.267	0.246	0.229

70	0.533	0.467	0.415	0.373	0.340	0.311	0.287	0.267
80	0.609	0.533	0.474	0.427	0.388	0.356	0.328	0.305
90	0.636	0.600	0.533	0.480	0.436	0.400	0.369	0.343
100	0.762	0.667	0.593	0.533	0.485	0.445	0.410	0.381

Dose (mcg/kg/min) = CF × Rate (mL/hr).

Calculation Factors (CF) by Patient Weight (35-70 kg) for Levophed 4 mg/250 mL

kg	35	40	45	50	55	60	65	70
CF	0.0076	0.0067	0.0059	0.0053	0.0048	0.0044	0.0041	0.0038

Norepinephrine (Levophed)

Norepinephrine (Levophed)

**Norepinephrine (Levophed) Drip Rate Calculation Chart—
Patient Weight 75-110 kg (165-242 lbs)**
Concentration: 16 mcg/mL (1 amp/250 mL)

| lbs | 165 | 176 | 189 | 199 | 209 | 220 | 231 | 242 |
kg	75	80	85	90	95	100	105	110
mL/hr				Dose = mcg/kg/min				
5	0.018	0.016	0.015	0.015	0.014	0.013	0.013	0.012
10	0.035	0.033	0.031	0.030	0.028	0.027	0.025	0.024
15	0.055	0.050	0.047	0.044	0.042	0.040	0.038	0.036
20	0.071	0.067	0.063	0.059	0.056	0.053	0.051	0.049
25	0.089	0.084	0.078	0.074	0.070	0.066	0.063	0.060
30	0.107	0.100	0.094	0.089	0.084	0.080	0.076	0.073
35	0.124	0.116	0.110	0.103	0.098	0.093	0.089	0.085
40	0.142	0.133	0.126	0.119	0.112	0.107	0.102	0.097
45	0.160	0.150	0.141	0.133	0.126	0.120	0.114	0.109
50	0.178	0.167	0.157	0.148	0.140	0.133	0.127	0.121
55	0.195	0.183	0.172	0.163	0.154	0.146	0.139	0.133
60	0.213	0.200	0.188	0.178	0.168	0.160	0.152	0.146

70	0.249	0.233	0.220	0.207	0.196	0.187	0.178	0.170
80	0.284	0.267	0.251	0.237	0.225	0.213	0.203	0.194
90	0.320	0.300	0.282	0.267	0.253	0.240	0.229	0.218
100	0.356	0.338	0.314	0.296	0.281	0.267	0.254	0.242

Dose (mcg/kg/min) = CF × Rate (mL/hr).

Calculation Factors (CF) by Patient Weight (75-110 kg) for Levophed 4 mg/250 mL

kg	75	80	85	90	95	100	105	110
CF	0.0036	0.0033	0.0031	0.0029	0.0028	0.0027	0.0025	0.0024

Norepinephrine (Levophed)

Octreotide (Sandostatin)

USES
For the treatment of acute esophageal and upper GI hemorrhage.

SOLUTION PREPARATION
An octreotide drip is prepared by adding 1200 mcg (2.4 mL of 500 mcg/mL) Sandostatin to 250 mL of 0.9% NaCl or D5W. **Final concentration:** 1200 mcg/ 250 mL (4.8 mcg/mL).

DOSE
Initial bolus dose IV is 50-250 mcg, followed by continuous infusion of 50-250 mcg/hr (10-50 mL/hr of standard solution). Usual dose is 1200 mcg over 24 hours, or 50 mcg/hr.

WARNINGS
Hypoglycemia or hyperglycemia may occur during infusion; obtain blood sugars as needed.

ADVERSE REACTIONS
Nausea, diarrhea, abdominal pain, vomiting, headache; generally well tolerated, with few adverse effects.

INCOMPATIBILITY
None specified. Because of lack of data, this drug should not be mixed with other medications except as noted below.

COMPATIBILITY
Heparin   TPN

NURSING CONSIDERATIONS
1. Consult the Octreotide Drip Rate Calculation Chart to determine the drip rate.
2. Octreotide should be administered via an IV pump to ensure controlled infusion.
3. Closely monitor hemoglobin and hematocrit to observe signs of efficacy and decreased GI bleeding.

Octreotide (Sandostatin) Drip Rate Calculation Chart
Octreotide (Sandostatin) 1200 mcg in 250 mL (Concentration: 4.8 mcg/mL)

Dose	Infusion rate
50 mcg/hr	10 mL/hr
100 mcg/hr	20 mL/hr
150 mcg/hr	30 mL/hr
200 mcg/hr	40 mL/hr

Octreotide (Sandostatin)

Pantoprazole (Protonix)

USES

Pantoprazole is used to treat acute GI bleeding, duodenal or gastric ulcers, and severe erosive esophagitis. The IV dosage form is used for patients who are unable to take the oral tablets.

SOLUTION PREPARATION

Mix 40-mg vial with 10 mL of diluent from 100-mL infusion bag of D5W or NS and swirl vial gently. Do not shake. **Final concentration:** 0.4 mg/mL. The 80-mg dose is prepared by taking two 40-mg vials and adding 10 ml of diluent (NS or D5W) to each, and then adding the contents of each vial to 80 ml of final solution. Final concentration is 80 mg/100 mL or 0.8 mg/mL. Alternatively, after reconstitution, bolus doses of 40-80 mg may be given IV over 2 minutes using a syringe pump and a 1.2-micron filter.

DOSE

The usual IV bolus dose is 40 mg per day. Doses of 40 mg twice daily also may be used. For Zollinger-Ellison syndrome, 80 mg every 12 hours may be used. For patients in ICU and with severe GI bleeding, a 40-80 mg loading dose, followed by 8 mg/hr by continuous infusion may be used. Daily doses in excess of 240 mg have not been studied and are not recommended. The original formulation of pantoprazole needed to be filtered with a 1.2-micron in-line filter, but the newest version does not.

WARNINGS

1. Should only be given by IV infusion, not IM or SC.
2. IV doses should be switched to oral tablets (40 mg) as soon as possible.
3. May precipitate after mixing final solution; therefore filtration is required at the time of administration.
4. Use caution in patients with severe hepatic impairment. The elimination half-life is prolonged and some accumulation may occur.

ADVERSE REACTIONS

Generally mild and infrequent. Pantoprazole is usually well tolerated, but rarely the following symptoms may be noted:
1. Abdominal pain
2. Headache
3. Confusion
4. Diarrhea

INCOMPATIBILITY

A single dedicated line is usually preferred. The line should be flushed with D5W, NS, or LR.

COMPATIBILITY

No known documented. Protonix should not be infused with other drug infusions.

NURSING CONSIDERATIONS

1. Refrigerate any unused drug vials until mixed.
2. Monitor pain levels; concomitant antacids may be indicated.

Pantoprazole (Protonix)

Pantoprazole (Protonix) Drip Rate Calculation Chart
(Final Concentrations: 40 mg/100 mL [0.4 mg/mL] or 80 mg/100 mL [0.8 mg/mL])

Bolus doses		Infusion dose
40 mg in 100 mL Infuse over 30 min	80 mg in 100 mL Infuse over 30 min	8 mg/hr (80 mg/100 mL)
200 mL/hr	200 mL/hr	Set infusion at 10 mL/hr

Phenylephrine (Neo-Synephrine)

USES
1. Treatment of vascular failure in shock, shock-like state, drug-induced hypotension, or hypersensitivity.
2. To overcome paroxysmal supraventricular tachycardia.

SOLUTION PREPARATION
A phenylephrine infusion is prepared by adding 10 mg (one ampule) phenylephrine to 250 mL D5W or NS. **Final concentration:** 10 mg/250 mL (40 mcg/mL). Do not use if solution is brown in color or precipitate is present.

DOSE
The usual initial dose is 100-180 mcg/min. When BP is stabilized, a maintenance dose of 40-60 mcg/min usually suffices.

WARNINGS
1. Blood volume depletion should be corrected before phenylephrine therapy is instituted.
2. Extravasation or peripheral ischemia can cause sloughing and necrosis of tissue in the surrounding area. ***Antidote:*** The site should be infiltrated with a 10-mL solution containing 5 mg phentolamine (Regitine); a fine hypodermic needle should be used.
3. Phenylephrine contains sodium metabisulfite; use with caution in patients with sulfite sensitivity.
4. Use with caution in elderly patients and patients with hyperthyroidism, bradycardia, partial heart block, myocardial disease, or arteriosclerosis.
5. Halogenated hydrocarbon anesthetics may sensitize myocardium to the effects of phenylephrine leading to serious arrhythmias.
6. Oxytocic drugs may potentiate the pressor effect of phenylephrine.

ADVERSE REACTIONS
Headache, reflex bradycardia, excitability, restlessness, and (rarely) arrhythmias.

INCOMPATIBILITY

Nitroglycerin
Nitroprusside
Phenytoin

Propofol
Thiopental

COMPATIBILITY

Amiodarone
Chloramphenicol
Cisatracurium
Dobutamine
Etomidate
Famotidine
Haloperidol

Inamrinone
Levofloxacin
Lidocaine
Potassium chloride
Remifentanil
Sodium bicarbonate
Zidovudine

NURSING CONSIDERATIONS

1. Consult the Phenylephrine Drip Rate Calculation Chart to determine the drip rate.
2. Except in cardiac arrest situations, phenylephrine should be administered via an IV pump to ensure controlled infusion.
3. The patient's BP should be monitored every 5 minutes from the time the phenylephrine infusion is started until the desired effect is achieved, then every 15 minutes while the drug is being infused.
4. Closely document changes in skin color or temperature in the extremities as a monitor for ischemia. Observe patients for extravasation. Closely document changes in HR, renal output, and ECG.

Phenylephrine (Neo-Synephrine)

Phenylephrine (Neo-Synephrine) Drip Rate Calculation Chart
Phenylephrine 10 mg in 250 mL (Concentration: 40 mcg/mL)

Dose	Infusion rate
40 mcg/min	60 mL/hr
50 mcg/min	75 mL/hr
60 mcg/min	90 mL/hr
70 mcg/min	105 mL/hr
80 mcg/min	120 mL/hr
90 mcg/min	135 mL/hr
100 mcg/min	150 mL/hr
110 mcg/min	165 mL/hr
120 mcg/min	180 mL/hr
130 mcg/min	195 mL/hr
140 mcg/min	210 mL/hr
150 mcg/min	225 mL/hr
160 mcg/min	240 mL/hr
170 mcg/min	255 mL/hr
180 mcg/min	270 mL/hr

Procainamide (Pronestyl)

USES

1. Ventricular ectopy (premature ventricular contractions, ventricular tachycardia, ventricular fibrillation) after lidocaine has failed.
2. Treatment of atrial fibrillation or paroxysmal atrial tachycardia.
3. Treatment of arrhythmias that occur during surgery.

SOLUTION PREPARATION

A procainamide infusion is prepared by adding 1 g (one 1-g vial) procainamide to 250 mL D5W or NS. **Final concentration:** 1 g/250 mL (4 mg/mL). Can also mix 2 g in 500 mL D5W (4 mg/mL).

Solutions of procainamide that are darker than light amber or otherwise discolored should not be used.

DOSE

1. A loading dose of 50-100 mg every 5 minutes (rate not greater than 25-50 mg/min) until arrhythmia is controlled; adverse effects occur; or until 500 mg have been administered, after which it may be advisable to wait 10 minutes to allow distribution of the drug before additional doses are given. Alternatively, a loading dose of 500 mg over 30 minutes, up to 1-1.25 g over 1-1½ hours, may be given.
2. A continuous IV infusion of 1-6 mg/min is administered.

WARNINGS

1. Use with caution in patients with renal or liver disease or congestive heart failure (CHF).
2. Administer with caution in patients with an acute myocardial infarction (AMI) and organic heart disease.
3. Use with caution, if at all, in patients with marked disturbances of AV conduction. It is contraindicated in patients with complete heart block unless a pacemaker is operative.
4. Use with caution in patients with known sensitivity to sulfiting agents.

5. Possibility of cross-sensitivity between procainamide and procaine.
6. Use with caution, if at all, in patients with myasthenia gravis.
7. Use with caution in conjunction with neuromuscular blocking agents.
8. When administered with other antiarrhythmic agents, cardiac effects may be additive or antagonistic and toxic effects may be additive.

ADVERSE REACTIONS
1. Severe hypotension.
2. Atrioventricular conduction disturbances, premature ventricular contractions, ventricular tachycardia, ventricular fibrillation, and asystole.
3. Confusion.

INCOMPATIBILITY

Aminophylline	Diltiazem
Barbiturates	Esmolol
Bretylium	Ethacrynate
Inamrinone	Phenytoin
Magnesium sulfate	Sodium bicarbonate
Milrinone	

COMPATIBILITY

Amiodarone	Heparin
Atracurium	Hydrocortisone
Cisatracurium	Lidocaine
Diltiazem	Potassium chloride
Dobutamine	Ranitidine
Famotidine	Remifentanil
Flumazenil	Verapamil

NURSING CONSIDERATIONS
1. Consult the Procainamide Drip Rate Calculation Chart to determine the drip rate.
2. Except in cardiac arrest situations, procainamide should be administered via an IV pump to ensure controlled infusion.
3. The ECG should be monitored continuously and the BP checked at 2- to 3-minute intervals during

Procainamide (Pronestyl)

administration of the loading dose. If the QRS complex widens >50% and the PR interval is prolonged or BP drops >15 mm Hg, temporarily discontinue the drug.

4. Monitor the BP at the start of the IV infusion and with each increase in dose. After the desired results are obtained, monitor BP at least hourly and document. Any disproportionate rise or fall in BP should be reported to the physician.

5. Closely monitor and document changes in the patient's HR and the ECG.

Procainamide (Pronestyl) Drip Rate Calculation Chart
Procainamide 1 g in 250 mL (Concentration: 4 mg/mL)

Dose	Infusion rate
0.5 mg/min	8 mL/hr
1 mg/min	15 mL/hr
1.5 mg/min	23 mL/hr
2 mg/min	30 mL/hr
2.5 mg/min	38 mL/hr
3 mg/min	45 mL/hr
3.5 mg/min	53 mL/hr
4 mg/min	60 mL/hr
4.5 mg/min	68 mL/hr
5 mg/min	75 mL/hr
5.5 mg/min	83 mL/hr
6 mg/min	90 mL/hr

Procainamide (Pronestyl)

Propofol (Diprivan)

USES
1. Induction or maintenance of anesthesia for inpatients.
2. Sedation for the ICU or CSU patient.

SOLUTION PREPARATION
Premixed solutions are available as 10 mg/mL in 50-mL and 100-mL emulsions. Do not use if there is evidence of separation of phases of emulsion.

DOSE
1. Initial dose is 20 mcg/kg/min as slow IV infusion. Rapid bolus injection should be avoided and can result in hypotension, oxyhemoglobin desaturation, apnea, airway obstruction, or oxygen desaturation.
2. Maintenance infusion is 25-75 mcg/kg/min.

WARNINGS
1. An 80% reduction in dose should be considered for elderly or debilitated patients.
2. Avoid in patients with increased intracranial pressure or impaired cerebral circulation.
3. Avoid in children.
4. Abrupt discontinuation can result in rapid awakening, anxiety, agitation, and resistance to mechanical ventilation.

ADVERSE REACTIONS
1. *Incidence >10%:* Nausea.
2. *Incidence 1%-10%:* Fever, hypotension, bradycardia, apnea, vomiting, abdominal cramping, cough, flushing.
3. *Incidence 1%:* Chest pain, dry mouth, somnolence, tachycardia, syncope, agitation, bronchospasm, diarrhea, ear pain, pruritus, dyspnea, tremor, twitching.

INCOMPATIBILITY
Amikacin
Amphotericin B
Ascorbic acid

Atracurium
Atropine
Blood

Bretylium
Calcium chloride
Ciprofloxacin
Diazepam
Digoxin
Doxacurium
Doxorubicin
Gentamicin
Methotrexate
Methylprednisolone
Metoclopramide
Midazolam
Minocycline
Mitoxantrone
Pancuronium
Phenylephrine
Phenytoin
Plasma
Serum
Tobramycin
Verapamil

COMPATIBILITY

Acyclovir
Alfentanil
Aminophylline
Ampicillin
Aztreonam
Bumetanide
Buprenorphine
Butorphanol
Calcium gluconate
Carboplatin
Cefazolin
Cefotaxime
Cefotetan
Ceftazidime
Ceftizoxime
Ceftriaxone
Cefuroxime
Chlorpromazine
Cimetidine
Cisplatin
Clindamycin
Cyclophosphamide
Cyclosporine
Cytarabine
Dexamethasone
Diphenhydramine
Dobutamine
Dopamine
Doxycycline
Droperidol
Enalaprilat
Ephedrine
Epinephrine
Esmolol
Famotidine
Fentanyl
Fluconazole
Fluorouracil
Furosemide
Ganciclovir
Glycopyrrolate
Granisetron
Haloperidol
Heparin
Hydrocortisone
Hydromorphone
Hydroxyzine
Ifosfamide
Imipenem/cilastatin
Inamrinone
Insulin
Isoproterenol
Ketamine
Labetalol
Levorphanol
Lidocaine
Lorazepam
Magnesium sulfate
Mannitol
Meperidine
Midazolam
Milrinone

Propofol (Diprivan)

Morphine
Nafcillin
Nalbuphine
Naloxone
Nitroglycerin
Nitroprusside
Norepinephrine
Ofloxacin
Ondansetron
Paclitaxel
Pentobarbital
Phenobarbital
Phenylephrine
Piperacillin

Potassium chloride
Prochlorperazine
Propranolol
Ranitidine
Scopolamine
Sodium bicarbonate
Succinylcholine
Sufentanil
Thiopental
Ticarcillin
Ticarcillin/clavulanate
Vancomycin
Vecuronium

NURSING CONSIDERATIONS

1. Propofol colors the urine green.
2. Consult the Propofol Drip Rate Calculation Chart to determine the drip rate.
3. Except in cardiac arrest, propofol should be administered via an IV pump to ensure controlled infusion.
4. BP should be measured every 15 minutes until stable, then at least hourly as long as drip remains in use.
5. Cardiorespiratory functions should be monitored in all patients.
6. Daily monitoring of serum lipids is recommended, especially in patients receiving high doses for long periods.
7. Discard after 12 hours if administered directly from vial or after 6 hours if transferred to D5W minibag. Tubing also should be replaced every 12 hours to deter microbial contamination.
8. Target level of sedation is Ramsey score of 5. Document about every 4 hours. Perform a sedation holiday (a temporary dose reduction to assess neurologic and respiratory function) every day for patients on therapy for more than 48 hours.

Propofol (Diprivan) Drip Rate Calculation Chart
Propofol 50-mL Infusion Vials (Concentration: 10 mg/mL)
Common Infusion Rates (Usual Doses: 5-50 mcg/kg/min)

Patient weight (kg)	10 (mcg/kg/min)	20 (mcg/kg/min)	30 (mcg/kg/min)	40 (mcg/kg/min)
50	3 mL/hr	6 mL/hr	9 mL/hr	12 mL/hr
60	3.6 mL/hr	7.2 mL/hr	10.8 mL/hr	14.4 mL/hr
70	4.2 mL/hr	8.4 mL/hr	12.6 mL/hr	16.8 mL/hr
80	4.8 mL/hr	9.6 mL/hr	14.4 mL/hr	19.2 mL/hr
90	5.4 mL/hr	10.8 mL/hr	16.2 mL/hr	21.6 mL/hr
100	6 mL/hr	12 mL/hr	18 mL/hr	24 mL/hr

Dose (mcg/kg/min) = CF × Rate (mL/hr).
NOTE: Premixed 50 mL bottles should hang for 12 hours maximum; if transferred to evacuated bottle, then 6 hours maximum.

Calculation Factors (CF) by Patient Weight (45-100 kg) for 10 mg/mL Concentration

kg	45	50	55	60	65	70	75	80	85	90	95	100
CF	3.70	3.33	3.03	2.78	2.56	2.38	2.22	2.08	1.96	1.85	1.75	1.67

Propofol (Diprivan)

Reteplase (Retavase)

USES
As a thrombolytic for treatment of acute myocardial infarction (AMI) to improve ventricular function.

SOLUTION PREPARATION
Mix 10 units reteplase for IV push administration with the diluent, syringe, needle, and dispensing pin in the kit. Swirl until it dissolves. Do not shake. A second 10-unit dose is included in the kit for use in 30 minutes.

DOSE
1. Usual dose is 10 units IV bolus over 2 minutes as soon as possible after onset of chest pain.
2. A second dose of 10 units is repeated in 30 minutes.

WARNINGS
1. Increased risk of bleeding, especially in the presence of anticoagulant drugs.
2. Heparin doses of 5000-unit bolus and 1000 units/hr or 800 units/hr for patients <80 kg may be used.
3. Administration of reteplase is contraindicated in cases of active internal bleeding; history of GI bleeding within 6 weeks; CVA within 2 years; thrombocytopenia; uncontrolled hypertension, intracranial neoplasm, arteriovenous malformations, or aneurysm; and history of severe allergic reactions to reteplase, tissue plasminogen activator (TPA), or streptokinase.

ADVERSE REACTIONS
1. Bleeding is the major side effect. Intracranial hemorrhage (0.8%) or stroke has been reported as a complication. Minor bleeding such as increased bruising, hematuria, GI bleeding, bleeding at the injection site (up to 48.6%), and hematemesis are possible.
2. Allergic reactions, anaphylaxis are rare.
3. Hypotension and arrhythmias are possible (>10%).

INCOMPATIBILITY

All medications. Retavase should be administered in a separate IV line whenever possible and should not be mixed with any other medications.

COMPATIBILITY

None.

NURSING CONSIDERATIONS

1. Use a separate IV site; do not administer with heparin because of incompatibility.
2. Watch closely for bleeding or anaphylaxis.
3. Minimize arterial and venous punctures for at least 24 hours after administration.
4. Heparin and aspirin (160-325 mg) should be used with reteplase to reduce risk of rethrombosis.

Reteplase (Retavase)

Tenecteplase (TNKase)

USES
As a thrombolytic for treatment of acute myocardial infarction (AMI) to improve ventricular function.

SOLUTION PREPARATION
Add 10 mL of sterile water to the TNKase vial; gently swirl until it dissolves. Do not shake. Withdraw the desired recommended dose and administer via IV push.

Use solution immediately upon reconstitution. If not used immediately, store under refrigeration and use within 8 hours.

DOSE
Usual single bolus dose is up to 50 mg over 5 seconds based on patient weight. See the Tenecteplase Dosing Chart.

WARNINGS
1. Increased risk of bleeding, especially in the presence of anticoagulant drugs.
2. Heparin doses of 5000-unit bolus and 1000 units/hr or 800 units/hr for patients <80 kg may be used.
3. Administration of tenecteplase is contraindicated in cases of active internal bleeding, history of GI bleeding within 6 weeks, history of CVA, thrombocytopenia, uncontrolled hypertension (SBP >180 and/or DBP >110), intracranial or intraspinal surgery or trauma within 2 months, intracranial neoplasm, arteriovenous malformations or aneurysm, or known bleeding diathesis.
4. The risk of major bleeding complications is higher in patients >65 years of age. The incidence of intracranial hemorrhage and stroke is 0.4%-1% for patients <65 years of age, 1.6%-2.9% for patients aged 65-74 years, and 1.7%-3% for patients ≥75 years of age.

ADVERSE REACTIONS
1. Bleeding is the major side effect. Intracranial hemorrhage (0.9%) and stroke (1.8%) have been reported as complications. Minor bleeding, such

as increased bruising, hematuria, GI bleeding, hematoma (12.3%), bleeding at the injection site, and hematemesis, is possible.
2. Allergic reactions, anaphylaxis are rare.
3. Hypotension and arrhythmias are possible (>10%).

INCOMPATIBILITY
All dextrose solutions

COMPATIBILITY
Normal saline

NURSING CONSIDERATIONS
1. Use a separate IV site; do not administer with any dextrose-containing solutions because of incompatibility.
2. Watch closely for bleeding or anaphylaxis.
3. Minimize arterial and venous punctures for at least 24 hours after administration.
4. Heparin (bolus dose 4000-5000 units, followed by continuous infusion of 800-1000 units/hr) and aspirin (160-325 mg) should be used with tenecteplase to reduce risk of rethrombosis.

Tenecteplase (TNKase)

Tenecteplase (TNKase) Dosing Chart
Acute Myocardial Infarction—TNKase 50 mg Added to 10 mL Sterile Water
(Concentration: 5.0 mg/mL)

Patient weight	Single loading dose over 5 sec	Volume of TNKase
<60 kg	30 mg	6 mL
60-69 kg	35 mg	7 mL
70-79 kg	40 mg	8 mL
80-89 kg	45 mg	9 mL
≥90 kg	50 mg	10 mL

Tirofiban HCl (Aggrastat)

USES
1. A nonpeptide antagonist of the platelet glycoprotein (GP) IIb/IIIa receptor that inhibits platelet aggregation.
2. Aggrastat, in combination with heparin, is indicated for the treatment of acute coronary syndromes, including patients who are to be managed medically and those undergoing PTCA or atherectomy.

SOLUTION PREPARATION
Add 25 mL (6.25 mg) tirofiban HCl to 100 mL NS or D5W to achieve a final concentration of 50 mcg/mL. Mix well before administration. Solution is good for 24 hours. Alternatively, withdraw and discard 50 mL from a 250-mL bag of sterile 0.9% NaCl or D5W and replace this volume with 50 mL of Aggrastat (from a 50-mL vial) to achieve a final concentration of 50 mcg/mL. A premixed 250-mL or 500-mL bag is available and also can be used.

DOSE
Usual dose is 0.4 mcg/kg/min for 30 minutes, then continued at 0.1 mcg/kg/min. Alternatively, accelerated dosing is 10 mcg/kg over 3 minutes and 0.15 mcg/kg/min infusion.

Onset of action is quick and dramatic because it will inhibit >90% of platelets by the end of the 30-minute infusion. Platelet aggregation inhibition is reversible following cessation of the infusion of tirofiban HCl.

Patients with severe renal insufficiency (i.e., creatinine clearance <30 mL/min) should receive half the usual rate of infusion. See the Tirofiban HCl Dosing Chart.

WARNINGS
1. Bleeding is the most common complication encountered during therapy with tirofiban HCl.
2. Most major bleeding occurs at the arterial access site for cardiac catheterization.

3. Use with caution in patients with platelet count <150,000/mm^3.
4. Use with caution in patients with hemorrhagic retinopathy.
5. Caution should be employed when tirofiban HCl is used with other drugs that affect hemostasis.
6. During therapy with tirofiban HCl, patients should be monitored for potential bleeding. When bleeding cannot be controlled with pressure, infusion of tirofiban HCl and heparin should be discontinued.

ADVERSE REACTIONS

The most common adverse effect is bleeding.

INCOMPATIBILITY

Diazepam (Valium)

COMPATIBILITY

Atropine
Dobutamine
Dopamine
Epinephrine
Famotidine
Furosemide
Heparin
Lidocaine
Midazolam
Morphine
Nitroglycerin
Potassium chloride
Propranolol

NURSING CONSIDERATIONS

1. Check patient's ACT, aPTT, and platelet count at baseline, then check within 6 hours after loading infusion and at least daily thereafter during therapy.
2. If patient experiences a platelet decrease to <90,000/mm^3, additional platelet counts should be performed to exclude pseudothrombocyto-penia. If thrombocytopenia is confirmed, tirofiban HCl and heparin should be discontinued.
3. In PTCA, before pulling the sheath, heparin should be discontinued for 3-4 hours and ACT <180 seconds or aPTT <45 seconds should be documented.

Tirofiban HCl (Aggrastat)

Tirofiban HCl (Aggrastat)

Tirofiban HCl (Aggrastat) Dosing Chart

| Patient weight | Normal renal function doses | | Creatinine clearance <30 | |
	30-min loading infusion rate	Maintenance infusion rate	30-min loading infusion rate	Maintenance infusion rate
30-37 kg	16 mL/hr	4 mL/hr	8 mL/hr	2 mL/hr
38-45 kg	20 mL/hr	5 mL/hr	10 mL/hr	3 mL/hr
46-54 kg	24 mL/hr	6 mL/hr	12 mL/hr	3 mL/hr
55-62 kg	28 mL/hr	7 mL/hr	14 mL/hr	4 mL/hr
63-70 kg	32 mL/hr	8 mL/hr	16 mL/hr	4 mL/hr
71-79 kg	36 mL/hr	9 mL/hr	18 mL/hr	5 mL/hr
80-87 kg	40 mL/hr	10 mL/hr	20 mL/hr	5 mL/hr
88-95 kg	44 mL/hr	11 mL/hr	22 mL/hr	6 mL/hr
96-104 kg	48 mL/hr	12 mL/hr	24 mL/hr	6 mL/hr
105-112 kg	52 mL/hr	13 mL/hr	26 mL/hr	7 mL/hr
113-120 kg	56 mL/hr	14 mL/hr	28 mL/hr	7 mL/hr
121-128 kg	60 mL/hr	15 mL/hr	30 mL/hr	8 mL/hr
129-137 kg	64 mL/hr	16 mL/hr	32 mL/hr	8 mL/hr
138-145 kg	68 mL/hr	17 mL/hr	34 mL/hr	9 mL/hr

Tirofiban HCl Injection (Aggrastat) Dosing Chart
*Bolus 10 mcg/kg Over 3 Minutes, 0.15 mcg/kg/min Infusion—
Accelerated Aggrastat Dosing
6.25 mg/125 mL (Final Concentration: 50 mcg/mL)*

| Patient weight range | | | |
lbs	kg	Bolus (over 3 min) volume (mL)	Maintenance infusion rate
95-109	43-49.9	9.3 (186 mL/hr × 3 min)	8 mL/hr
110-122	50-55.9	10.6 (212 mL/hr × 3 min)	10 mL/hr
123-138	56-62.9	12 (240 mL/hr × 3 min)	11 mL/hr
139-153	63-69.9	13.3 (266 mL/hr × 3 min)	12 mL/hr
154-168	70-76.9	14.7 (294 mL/hr × 3 min)	13 mL/hr
169-184	77-83.9	16.1 (322 mL/hr × 3 min)	14 mL/hr
185-199	84-90.9	17.5 (350 mL/hr × 3 min)	16 mL/hr
200-215	91-97.9	18.9 (378 mL/hr × 3 min)	17 mL/hr
216-228	98-103.9	20.2 (404 mL/hr × 3 min)	18 mL/hr
229-241	104-109.9	21.4 (428 mL/hr × 3 min)	19 mL/hr
242-254	110-115.9	22.6 (452 mL/hr × 3 min)	20 mL/hr
255-270	116-122.9	23.9 (478 mL/hr × 3 min)	22 mL/hr
271-285	123-129.9	25.3 (506 mL/hr × 3 min)	23 mL/hr
286-300	130-136.9	26.7 (534 mL/hr × 3 min)	24 mL/hr

Tirofiban HCl (Aggrastat)

Vasopressin (Pitressin)

USES

For the treatment of acute esophageal and upper GI hemorrhage. *Unapproved use:* For adult shock-refractory ventricular fibrillation (class IIB) as an alternative to epinephrine to support blood pressure.

SOLUTION PREPARATION

A vasopressin drip is prepared by adding 250 units (12.5 mL of 20 units/mL) vasopressin to 250 mL 0.9% NaCl or D5W. **Final concentration:** 250 units/250 mL (1 unit/mL).

DOSE

1. Initial infusion is started at 0.2 units/min and increased hourly as needed to a maximum rate of 1 unit/min.
2. During cardiac arrest, vasopressin 40 units IV may be given as a single bolus dose to support blood pressure.

WARNINGS

1. Anaphylaxis and/or shock have occurred shortly after beginning infusion; discontinue infusion if either of these occurs.
2. Vasopressin may produce a reduction in cardiac function, decreased cardiac output, myocardial contractility, and decreased coronary blood flow. Use with caution in patients with cardiovascular diseases.
3. May cause angina. (Concurrent nitroglycerin administration may decrease cardiotoxic effect of vasopressin.)
4. Vasopressin may cause infarction or ischemia; gastric infarction, ischemic colitis, scrotal ischemia, cutaneous gangrene, and mottling and cyanosis of extremities, though rare, have been reported.

ADVERSE REACTIONS

1. *Cardiovascular:* Angina, bradycardia, hypertension, arrhythmias, peripheral vascular constriction, anaphylaxis.
2. *GI:* Abdominal cramps, gas, nausea, vomiting, diarrhea, ischemic colitis.
3. *Hypersensitivity:* Urticaria, angioedema, broncho-constriction, fever, rash, wheezing, dyspnea, circulatory collapse, anaphylaxis.
4. *Other:* Pallor, sweating, tremor, pounding in the head, vertigo, uterine cramps.

INCOMPATIBILITY

None specified. Because of the lack of available data, this drug should not be mixed with other medications.

NURSING CONSIDERATIONS

1. Consult the Vasopressin Drip Rate Calculation Chart to determine the drip rate.
2. Vasopressin should be administered via an IV pump to ensure controlled infusion.
3. Closely monitor and document changes in BP, HR, or in the rhythm strip. The patient's BP should be monitored every 5 minutes for the first hour and then hourly.
4. Closely monitor and document changes in skin color and other dermal changes.
5. Contact physician if any new onset of chest pain or abdominal pain occurs during vasopressin infusion.

Vasopressin (Pitressin)

Vasopressin (Pitressin)

Vasopressin (Pitressin) Drip Rate Calculation Chart
Vasopressin 250 units in 250 mL (Concentration: 1 unit/mL)

Dose	Infusion rate
0.2 units/min	12 mL/hr
0.3 units/min	18 mL/hr
0.4 units/min	24 mL/hr
0.5 units/min	30 mL/hr
0.6 units/min	36 mL/hr
0.7 units/min	42 mL/hr
0.8 units/min	48 mL/hr
0.9 units/min	54 mL/hr
1 units/min	60 mL/hr

ACLS Guidelines for Adult Emergency Cardiac Care Algorithms

Pulseless Ventricular Tachycardia (VT)/Ventricular Fibrillation (VF)

Basic life support	**Perform Primary ABCD Survey** • Correct critical problems *immediately* as they are identified. • Assess responsiveness. • Call for help/Call for defibrillator. *Airway* • Open the airway. *Breathing* • Deliver two slow breaths; administer oxygen as soon as it is available. *Circulation* • Perform chest compressions. *Defibrillation* • Ensure availability of monitor/defibrillator. • On arrival of AED/monitor/defibrillator, evaluate cardiac rhythm. • If PEA or asystole, continue CPR and go to appropriate algorithm. • If pulseless VF/VT, shock up to three times (200 J, 200-300 J, 360 J, or equivalent biphasic energy). ▼

Reevaluate Cardiac Rhythm
- If persistent or recurrent pulseless VF/VT, continue CPR and perform secondary ABCD survey.
- If PEA or asystole, continue CPR and go to appropriate algorithm.
- If return of spontaneous circulation:
- Assess vital signs.
- Maintain open airway.
- Provide ventilation; administer medications appropriate for rhythm, BP, and heart rate.

Advanced life support

Perform Secondary ABCD Survey
Airway
- Reassess effectiveness of initial airway maneuvers and interventions.
- Perform invasive airway management.

Pattern becomes CPR-drug-shock or CPR-drug-shock-shock-shock

Breathing
- Assess ventilation.
- Confirm ET tube placement (or other airway device) by at least two methods.

Continued

- Provide positive pressure ventilation/Evaluate effectiveness of ventilations.
- Secure airway device in place with commercial tube holder (preferred) or tape.

▼

Circulation
- Establish IV access and administer appropriate medications.

▼

Differential Diagnosis
- Search for and treat reversible causes.

▼

Epinephrine (Class Indeterminate)—1 mg (1:10,000 solution) IV every 3-5 minutes. (ET dose 2.0-2.5 mg diluted in 10-mL NS or distilled water.)
or
Vasopressin (Class IIb)—40 units IV bolus (administer only once). (If no response to vasopressin, may resume epinephrine after 10-20 minutes; epinephrine dose 1 mg every 3-5 minutes.)

▼

Defibrillate with 360 J (or equivalent biphasic energy) within 30-60 seconds.

▼

Consider antiarrhythmics (avoid use of multiple antiarrhythmics because of potential proarrhythmic effects).

- **Amiodarone** (Class IIb)—Initial bolus: 300 mg IV bolus diluted in 20-30 mL of NS or D5W. Consider repeat dose (150 mg IV bolus) in 3-5 minutes. If defibrillation successful, follow with 1 mg/min IV infusion for 6 hours (mix 900 mg in 500 mL NS), then decrease infusion rate to 0.5 mg/min IV infusion for 18 hours. Maximum daily dose 2.0 g IV/24 hr.
- **Lidocaine** (Class Indeterminate)—1.0-1.5 mg/kg IV bolus, consider repeat dose (0.5-0.75 mg/kg) in 5 minutes; maximum IV bolus dose 3 mg/kg. (The 1.5 mg/kg dose is recommended in cardiac arrest.) Endotracheal dose: 2-4 mg/kg. A single dose of 1.5 mg/kg is acceptable in cardiac arrest.
- **Magnesium** (Class IIb if hypomagnesemia present)—1-2 g IV (2-4 mL of a 50% solution) diluted in 10 mL of D5W if torsades de pointes or hypomagnesemia.
- **Procainamide** (Class IIb for recurrent pulseless VF/VT; class indeterminate for persistent pulseless VF/VT)—20 mg/min; maximum total dose 17 mg/kg.

Consider sodium bicarbonate 1 mEq/kg.

Modified from Aehlert B: *ACLS quick review study guide,* ed 2, St Louis, 2001, Mosby, pp 414-415.

Asystole

| Basic life support | **Perform Primary ABCD Survey**
• Correct critical problems *immediately* as they are identified.
• Assess responsiveness.
• Call for help/Call for defibrillator.

Airway
• Open the airway.

Breathing
• Deliver two slow breaths; administer oxygen as soon as it is available.

Circulation
• Perform chest compressions.

Defibrillation
• Ensure availability of monitor/defibrillator.
• On arrival of AED/monitor/defibrillator, perform secondary ABCD survey if rhythm is *not* pulseless VF/VT.

 |

- Scene survey—Documentation or other evidence of Do Not Attempt Resuscitation (DNAR)?
- Obvious signs of death? If yes, do not start/attempt resuscitation.

Advanced life support

Possible causes of asystole:
PATCH-4-MD
Pulmonary embolism
Acidosis
Tension pneumothorax
Cardiac tamponade
Hypovolemia (most common cause)

Perform Secondary ABCD Survey

Airway
- Reassess effectiveness of initial airway maneuvers and interventions.
- Perform invasive airway management.

Breathing
- Assess ventilation.
- Confirm ET tube placement (or other airway device) by at least two methods.
- Provide positive-pressure ventilation/Evaluate effectiveness of ventilations.
- Secure airway device in place with commercial tube holder (preferred) or tape.

Continued

ACLS Guidelines for Adult Emergency Cardiac Care Algorithms

Hypoxia
Heat/cold (hypothermia/ hyperthermia)
Hypokalemia/ hyperkalemia (and other electrolytes)
Myocardial infarction
Drug overdose/ accidents (cyclic antidepressants, calcium channel blockers, beta-blockers, digitalis)

Circulation
- Confirm presence of asystole (check lead/cable connections; ensure power to monitor is on, correct lead is selected, gain turned up; confirm asystole in second lead).
- Establish IV access and administer appropriate medications.

▼

Differential Diagnosis
- Search for and treat reversible causes (PATCH-4-MD).

▼

Consider immediate transcutaneous pacing.

▼

Epinephrine—1 mg (1:10,000 solution) IV every 3-5 minutes. (Endotracheal dose 2.0-2.5 mg diluted in 10 mL NS or distilled water.)

▼

Atropine—1 mg IV every 3-5 minutes to maximum 0.04 mg/kg (class IIb) (ET dose 2-3 mg diluted in 10 mL NS or distilled water).

▼

Consider **sodium bicarbonate** 1 mEq/kg:
- Known pre-existing hyperkalemia (class 1)
- Cyclic antidepressant overdose (IIa)
- To alkalinize urine in aspirin or other drug overdoses (IIa)
- Patient that has been intubated for one long arrest interval (IIb)
- On return of spontaneous circulation if long arrest interval (IIb)

▼

Consider termination of efforts:
- Evaluate the quality of the resuscitation attempt.
- Evaluate the resuscitation of atypical clinical features (e.g., hypothermia, reversible therapeutic or illicit drug use).
- Does support for cease-effort protocols exist?

Modified from Aehlert B: *ACLS quick review study guide,* ed 2, St Louis, 2001, Mosby, p 417.

Pulseless Electrical Activity (PEA)

Basic life support	**Perform Primary ABCD Survey** • Correct critical problems *immediately* as they are identified. • Assess responsiveness. • Call for help/Call for defibrillator. *Airway* • Open the airway. *Breathing* • Deliver two slow breaths; administer oxygen as soon as it is available. *Circulation* • Perform chest compressions. *Defibrillation* • Ensure availability of monitor/defibrillator. • On arrival of AED/monitor/defibrillator, perform secondary ABCD survey if rhythm is not pulseless VF/VT. ▼

Advanced life support	Perform Secondary ABCD Survey

Advanced life support

Possible causes of PEA: **PATCH-4-MD**
Pulmonary embolism
Acidosis
Tension pneumothorax
Cardiac tamponade
Hypovolemia (most common cause)
Hypoxia
Heat/cold (hypothermia/ hyperthermia)
Hypokalemia/ hyperkalemia (and other electrolytes)

Perform Secondary ABCD Survey

Airway
- Reassess effectiveness of initial airway maneuvers and interventions.
- Perform invasive airway management.

Breathing
- Assess ventilation.
- Confirm ET tube placement (or other airway device) by at least two methods.
- Provide positive-pressure ventilation/Evaluate effectiveness of ventilations.
- Secure airway device in place with commercial tube holder (preferred) or tape.

Circulation
- Establish IV access.
- Assess blood flow with Doppler. (If blood flow detected with Doppler, treat using hypotension/shock algorithm.)
- Administer appropriate medications.

Continued

Myocardial infarction
Drug overdose/ accidents (cyclic antidepressants, calcium channel blockers, beta-blockers, digitalis)

*D*ifferential Diagnosis
- Search for and treat reversible causes (PATCH-4-MD). (Fast narrow QRS—consider hypovolemia, tamponade, pulmonary embolism, tension pneumothorax; slow wide QRS—consider cyclic antidepressant overdose, calcium channel blocker, beta-blocker, or digitalis toxicity.)

Epinephrine—1 mg (1:10,000 solution) IV every 3-5 minutes. (Endotracheal dose 2-2.5 mg diluted in 10 mL NS or distilled water.)

▼

Atropine (if the rate is slow)—1 mg IV every 3-5 minutes to max 0.04 mg/kg (class IIb). (Endotracheal dose 2-3 mg diluted in 10 mL NS or distilled water.)

▼

Consider sodium bicarbonate 1 mEq/kg:
- Known preexisting hyperkalemia (class 1)
- Cyclic antidepressant overdose (IIa)
- To alkalinize urine in aspirin or other drug overdoses (IIa)

- Patient that has been intubated + long arrest interval (IIb)
- On return of spontaneous circulation if long arrest interval (IIb)

Consider termination of efforts.

Modified from Aehlert B: *ACLS quick review study guide,* ed 2, St Louis, 2001, Mosby, p 420.

Pulseless Electrical Activity (PEA): Clinical Signs and Treatment

Cause	Typical ECG findings	History, physical findings	Management
Mechanical causes Tension pneumothorax	Narrow QRS complex, slow rate (because of hypoxia)	History (trauma, asthma, ventilator, COPD). Unequal breath sounds, no pulse with CPR, neck vein distention, tracheal deviation, difficult to ventilate patient, hyper-resonance to percussion on affected side	Needle decompression—second intercostal space, midclavicular line
Cardiac tamponade	Narrow QRS complex, rapid rate (impending tamponade)—deteriorating to sudden bradycardia as terminal event	History (trauma, renal failure thoracic malignancy), no pulse with CPR, neck vein distention	Pericardiocentesis
Decreased preload Hypovolemia	Narrow QRS complex, rapid rate	History, flat neck veins	Volume replacement; find source (e.g., bleeding) and manage

		History	Volume replacement, antibiotics
Sepsis			
Massive pulmonary embolism	Narrow QRS complex, rapid rate	History, no pulse with CPR, neck vein distention, deep vein thrombosis in lower extremities	Pulmonary arteriogram, surgical embolectomy, fibrinolytics
Myocardial dysfunction			
Massive myocardial infarction	Q waves, ST segment changes, T wave inversion	History, ECG, enzyme levels	Emergency PTCA; if unavailable, fibrinolytics
Drug overdose			
Calcium channel blocker	Slow rate, prolonged PR interval, possible AV block	History of ingestion, empty bottles at the scene, check pupils, neurologic exam	Calcium IV, pacing
Beta-blocker	Slow rate, prolonged PR interval, possible AV block		Glucagon IV, pacing
Cyclic antidepressants	Rapid rate, prolonged QT interval, widening of QRS, ST segment changes		Sodium bicarbonate IV

Continued

ACLS Guidelines for Adult Emergency Cardiac Care Algorithms

Pulseless Electrical Activity (PEA): Clinical Signs and Treatment—cont'd

Cause	Typical ECG findings	History, physical findings	Management
Drug overdose—cont'd Digoxin	Slow rate, prolonged PR interval, shortened QT interval, T wave inversion or flattening		Fab antibodies
Electrolytes Hypokalemia	ST segment depression, T waves flatten, prominent U waves, QRS widens (uncommon in adults)	Prolonged diuretic therapy; administration of K^+ deficient parenteral fluids; severe GI fluid losses from gastric suctioning or lavage; prolonged vomiting or diarrhea, or laxative abuse without K^+ replacement	Rapid, controlled potassium infusion

Condition	ECG Findings	Causes	Treatment
Hyperkalemia	Rapid rate; tall, narrow, peaked (tented) T waves; QRS widens; flattened or absent P waves; ST segment elevation	History of acute or chronic renal failure; diabetes; dialysis fistulas; medications; severe cell damage such as from burns, trauma, crush injuries	Calcium chloride IV push (immediate); then combination of insulin, glucose, sodium bicarbonate; then sodium polystyrene sulfonate/sorbitol; dialysis (long-term)
Hypocalcemia	Prolonged QT internal and ST segment; VT, torsades de pointes	Acute or chronic renal failure, acute pancreatitis	Calcium chloride IV
Hypercalcemia	Shortened QT interval	Excessive intake of Ca^{++} supplements, prolonged immobility, thiazide diuretics	Magnesium sulfate, potassium, diuretics
Hypomagnesemia	Flattened T waves, slightly widened QRS complex, diminished voltage of P waves and QRS complexes, prominent U waves	Severe GI fluid losses from gastric suctioning or lavage, prolonged vomiting or diarrhea, or laxative abuse; administration of IV fluids or TPN without magnesium replacement; cancer chemotherapy	

Continued

Pulseless Electrical Activity (PEA): Clinical Signs and Treatment—cont'd

Cause	Typical ECG findings	History, physical findings	Management
Hypothermia Hypothermia	Initial tachycardia, then progressive bradycardia; J or Osborne waves	History of cold exposure, core body temperature	Rewarming guided by core temperature
Pulmonary causes Severe respiratory insufficiency/arrest resulting in hypoxia	Slow rate because of hypoxia	Cyanosis, blood gas results, airway obstruction	Ventilation
Postdefibrillation PEA After reversal of prolonged VF with electrical counter-shock			No specific intervention

Modified from Aehlert B: *ACLS quick review study guide,* ed 2, St Louis, 2001, Mosby, pp 422-423.

Basic life support	**Perform Primary ABCD Survey** • Correct critical problems *immediately* as they are identified. • Assess responsiveness. • Call for help/Call for defibrillator. *Airway* • Open the airway. *Breathing* • Deliver two slow breaths; administer oxygen as soon as it is available. *Circulation* • Perform chest compressions. *Defibrillation* • Ensure availability of monitor/defibrillator.

Continued

Advanced life support	**Perform Secondary ABCD Survey**
	• Administer oxygen, establish IV access, attach cardiac monitor, administer fluids as needed (O_2, IV, monitor, fluids).
	• Assess vital signs, attach pulse oximeter, and monitor BP.
	• Obtain and review 12-lead ECG, portable chest x-ray film.
	• Perform a focused history and physical exam.
	▼
	Identify the Patient's Cardiac Rhythm
	Is the patient experiencing serious signs and symptoms because of the bradycardia?
	• *Signs:* Low BP, shock, pulmonary congestion, congestive heart failure, angina, acute myocardial infarction (MI), ventricular ectopy
	• *Symptoms:* Chest pain, weakness, fatigue, dizziness, lightheadedness, shortness of breath, exercise intolerance, decreased level of responsiveness
	• If no serious signs and symptoms are present, observe.
	• If serious signs and symptoms are present, further intervention depends on the cardiac rhythm identified.

Is the QRS Narrow or Wide?

Narrow QRS bradycardia
- Sinus bradycardia
- Junctional rhythm
- Second-degree AV block, type 1
- Third-degree (complete) AV block

Medication Dosing

Narrow QRS bradycardia
- **Atropine IV**—0.5-1.0 mg IV; may repeat every 3-5 minutes to a total dose of 2.5 mg (0.03-0.04 mg/kg); total cumulative dose should not exceed 2.5 mg over 2.5 hours
- Transcutaneous pacemaker—Pacing should not be delayed while waiting for IV access or for atropine to take effect
- **Dopamine infusion**—5-10 mcg/kg/min
- **Epinephrine infusion**—2-10 mcg/min
- **Isoproterenol infusion**—2-10 mcg/min (low dose)

Wide QRS bradycardia
- Second-degree AV block, type II
- Third degree (complete) AV block
- Ventricular escape (idioventricular) rhythm

Wide QRS bradycardia
- Transcutaneous pacemaker—As an interim device until transvenous pacing can be accomplished
- **Dopamine infusion**: 5-20 mcg/kg/min
- **Epinephrine infusion**: 2-10 mcg/min
- **Isoproterenol infusion**: 2-10 mcg/min (low doses)

Modified from Aehlert B: *ACLS quick review study guide,* ed 2, St Louis, 2001, Mosby, p 430.

ACLS Guidelines for Adult Emergency Cardiac Care Algorithms

Narrow QRS Tachycardia

Basic life support

Perform Primary ABCD Survey
- Correct critical problems *immediately* as they are identified.
- Assess responsiveness.
- Call for help/Call for defibrillator.

Airway
- Open the airway.

Breathing
- Deliver two slow breaths; administer oxygen as soon as it is available.

Circulation
- Perform chest compressions.

Defibrillation
- Ensure availability of monitor/defibrillator.

▼

Advanced life support

Perform Secondary ABCD Survey
- Administer oxygen, establish IV access, attach cardiac monitor, administer fluids as needed (O_2, IV, monitor, fluids).
- Assess vital signs, attach pulse oximeter, and monitor BP.

- Obtain and review 12-lead ECG, portable chest x-ray film.
- Perform a focused history and physical exam.

- Is the patient stable or unstable?
- Is the patient experiencing serious signs and symptoms because of the tachycardia?

Attempt to identify patient's cardiac rhythm using:
- 12-lead ECG, clinical information
- Vagal maneuvers

If needed, administer **adenosine** 6 mg rapid IV bolus over 1-3 seconds after 1-2 minutes:
- May repeat 12-mg dose in 1-2 minutes if needed.
- Follow each dose immediately with 20-mL IV flush of NS.
- Use of adenosine is relatively contraindicated in patients with asthma.
- Decrease dose in patients on dipyridamole (Persantine) or carbamazepine (Tegretol); consider increasing dose in patients taking theophylline or caffeine-containing preparations.

Identify the Patient's Cardiac Rhythm

Continued

Narrow QRS Tachycardia—cont'd

Stable Patient

Junctional tachycardia		Paroxysmal supraventricular tachycardia (PSVT) (includes AVNRT or AVRT)		Ectopic atrial tachycardia or multifocal atrial tachycardia (MAT)	
Normal cardiac function	**Impaired cardiac function***	**Normal cardiac function**	**Impaired cardiac function***	**Normal cardiac function**	**Impaired cardiac function***
Amiodarone (IIb) **or** Beta-blocker (indeterminate) or Ca^{++} channel blocker (indeterminate)	Amiodarone (IIb)	*Priority order:* Ca^{++} channel blocker (class I), beta-blocker (class I), Digoxin (IIb), sync cardioversion	*Priority order:* Sync cardioversion, digoxin (IIb), amiodarone (IIb), diltiazem (IIb)	Ca^{++} channel blocker (IIb) **or** beta-blocker (IIb) **or** amiodarone (IIb) **or** flecainide (IIb) **or** propafenone (IIb) **or** digoxin (indeterminate) **Cardioversion ineffective**	Amiodarone (IIb) **or** diltiazem (IIb) **or** digoxin (indeterminate) **Cardioversion ineffective**

Unstable Patient

If hemodynamically unstable PSVT, perform synchronized cardioversion: 50 J, 100 J, 200 J, 300 J, 360 J (or equivalent biphasic energy)

*Impaired cardiac function = ejection fraction <40% or congestive heart failure.

Medication Dosing

Amiodarone—150 mg IV over 10 minutes followed by an infusion of 1 mg/min for 6 hours and then a maintenance infusion of 0.5 mg/min. Repeat supplementary infusions of 150 mg as necessary for recurrent or resistant dysrhythmias. Maximum total daily dose 2 g.

Beta-blockers—*Esmolol:* 0.5 mg/kg over 1 minute, followed by a maintenance infusion at 50 mcg/kg/min for 4 minutes. If inadequate response, administer a second bolus of 0.5 mg/kg over 1 minute and increase maintenance infusion to 100 mcg/kg/min. The bolus dose (0.5 mg/kg) and titration of the maintenance infusion (addition of 50 mcg/kg/min) can be repeated every 4 minutes to a maximum infusion of 300 mcg/kg/min. *Metoprolol:* 5 mg slow IV push over 5 minutes × 3 as needed to a total dose of 15 mg over 15 minutes.

Calcium channel blockers—*Diltiazem:* 0.25 mg/kg over 2 minutes (e.g., 15-20 mg). If ineffective, 0.35 mg/kg over 2 minutes (e.g., 20-25 mg) in 15 minutes. Maintenance infusion 5-15 mg/hr, titrated to heart rate if chemical conversion successful. Calcium chloride (2-4 mg/kg) may be given **slow** IV push if borderline hypotension exists before administration. *Verapamil:* 2.5-5.0 mg slow IV push over 2 minutes. May repeat with 5-10 mg in 15-30 minutes. Maximum dose 20 mg.

Digoxin—Loading dose 10-15 mcg/kg lean body weight.

Flecainide, propafenone—IV form not currently approved for use in the United States.

Modified from Aehlert B: *ACLS quick review study guide,* ed 2, St Louis, 2001, Mosby, pp 435-436.

Continued

Narrow QRS Tachycardia—cont'd

Type of countershock	Dysrhythmia	Recommended energy levels
Defibrillation	Pulseless VF/VT	200 J, 200-300 J, 360 J or equivalent biphasic energy
	Sustained polymorphic VT	200 J, 200-300 J, 360 J or equivalent biphasic energy
	VT with a pulse	100 J, 200 J, 300 J, 360 J or equivalent biphasic energy
	Undue delay in delivery of synchronized countershock	Depends on rhythm
Synchronized cardioversion	Paroxysmal supraventricular tachycardia (PSVT)	50 J, 100 J, 200 J, 300 J, 360 J or equivalent biphasic energy
	Atrial flutter	50 J, 100 J, 200 J, 300 J, 360 J or equivalent biphasic energy
	Atrial fibrillation	100 J, 200 J, 300 J, 360 J or equivalent biphasic energy
	VT with a pulse	100 J, 200 J, 300 J, 360 J or equivalent biphasic energy

Modified from Aehlert B: *ACLS quick review study guide,* ed 2, St Louis, 2001, Mosby, p 436.

Atrial Fibrillation/Atrial Flutter Algorithm

| Basic life support | **Perform Primary ABCD Survey**
• Correct critical problems *immediately* as they are identified.
• Assess responsiveness.
• Call for help/Call for defibrillator.

Airway
• Open the airway.

Breathing
• Deliver two slow breaths; administer oxygen as soon as it is available.

Circulation
• Perform chest compressions.

Defibrillation
• Ensure availability of monitor/defibrillator.

 |

Continued

Atrial Fibrillation/Atrial Flutter Algorithm—cont'd

Advanced life support	**Perform Secondary ABCD Survey** • Administer oxygen, establish IV access, attach cardiac monitor, administer fluids as needed (O_2, IV, monitor, fluids). • Assess vital signs, attach pulse oximeter, and monitor BP. • Obtain and review 12-lead ECG, portable chest x-ray film. • Perform a focused history and physical exam. ▼ • Is the patient stable or unstable? • Is the patient's cardiac function normal or impaired? • Is the patient experiencing serious signs and symptoms because of the tachycardia? • Attempt to identify patient's cardiac rhythm using 12-lead ECG, clinical information. • Is Wolff-Parkinson-White syndrome (WPW) present? If yes, see WPW algorithm. • Has atrial fibrillation/atrial flutter been present for > or <48 hours? ▼ **Identify the Patient's Cardiac Rhythm**

Stable Patient			
Normal cardiac function		**Impaired cardiac function***	
Onset <48 hr Control rate	**Onset >48 hr Control rate**	**Onset <48 hr Control rate**	**Onset >48 hr Control rate**
Calcium channel blocker (class 1) **or** Beta-blocker (class 1) **or** Digoxin (IIb)	Calcium channel blocker (class 1) **or** Beta-blocker (class 1) **or** Digoxin (IIb)	Diltiazem (IIb) **or** Amiodarone (IIb) **or** Digoxin (IIb)	Diltiazem (IIb) **or** Amiodarone (IIb) **or** Digoxin (IIb)
Convert rhythm	**Convert rhythm**	**Convert rhythm**	**Convert rhythm**
Cardioversion **or** Amiodarone (IIa) **or** Procainamide (IIa) **or** Ibutilide (IIa) **or** Flecainide (IIa) **or** Propafenone (IIa)	Delayed cardioversion **or** Early cardioversion	Cardioversion **or** Amiodarone (IIb)	Delayed cardioversion **or** Early cardioversion

*Impaired cardiac function = ejection fraction <40% or congestive heart failure.

Continued

Delayed cardioversion: Anticoagulation therapy for 3 weeks before cardioversion, for at least 48 hours in conjunction with cardioversion, and for at least 4 weeks after successful cardioversion.

Early cardioversion: IV heparin immediately, transesophageal echocardiography (TEE) to rule out atrial thrombus, cardioversion within 24 hours, anticoagulation × 4 weeks.

Unstable Patient

If hemodynamically unstable, perform synchronized cardioversion:
- Atrial fibrillation: 100 J, 200 J, 300 J, 360 J, or equivalent biphasic energy
- Atrial flutter: 50 J, 100 J, 200 J, 300 J, 360 J, or equivalent biphasic energy

Medication Dosing

Amiodarone—150 mg IV bolus over 10 minutes followed by an infusion of 1 mg/min for 6 hours and then a maintenance infusion of 0.5 mg/min. Repeat supplementary infusions of 150 mg as necessary for recurrent or resistant dysrhythmias. Maximum total daily dose 2 g.

Beta-blockers—*Esmolol:* 0.5 mg/kg over 1 minute followed by a maintenance infusion at 50 mcg/kg/min for 4 minutes. If inadequate response, administer a second bolus of 0.5 mg/kg over 1 minute and increase maintenance infusion to 100 mcg/kg/min. The bolus dose (0.5 mg/kg) and titration of the maintenance infusion (addition of 50 mcg/kg/min) can be repeated every 4 minutes to a maximum infusion of 300 mcg/kg/min. *Metoprolol:* 5 mg slow IV push over 5 minutes × 3 as needed to a total dose of 15 mg over 15 minutes.

Propranolol: 0.1 mg/kg slow IV push divided in 3 equal doses at 2-3 minute intervals. Do not exceed 1 mg/min. Repeat after 2 minutes, if necessary. *Atenolol:* 5 mg slow IV (over 5 min). Wait 10 minutes, then give second dose of 5 mg slow IV (over 5 min).

Calcium channel blockers—*Diltiazem:* 0.25 mg/kg over 2 minutes (e.g., 15-20 mg). If ineffective, 0.35 mg/kg over 2 minutes (e.g., 20-25 mg) in 15 minutes. Maintenance infusions 5-15 mg/hr, titrated to heart rate if chemical conversion successful. Calcium chloride (2-4 mg/kg) may be given **slow** IV push if borderline hypotension exists before diltiazem administration. *Verapamil:* 2.5-5.0 mg slow IV push over 2 minutes. May repeat with 5-10 mg in 15-30 minutes. Maximum dose 20 mg.

Ibutilide—Adults ≥60 kg: 1 mg (10 mL) over 10 minutes. May repeat × 1 in 10 minutes. Adults <60 kg: 0.01 mg/kg IV over 10 minutes.

Procainamide—100 mg over 5 minutes (20 mg/min). Maximum total dose 17 mg/kg. Maintenance infusion 1-4 mg/min. *Flecainide propafenone:* IV form not currently approved for use in the United States.

Sotalol—1-1.5 mg/kg IV slowly at rate of 10 mg/min.

Modified from Aehlert B: *ACLS quick review study guide,* ed 2, St Louis, 2001, Mosby, p 438.

Wolff-Parkinson-White (WPW) Syndrome Algorithm

Basic life support	**Perform Primary ABCD Survey** • Correct critical problems immediately as they are identified. • Assess responsiveness. • Call for help/Call for defibrillator. *Airway* • Open the airway. *Breathing* • Deliver two slow breaths; administer oxygen as soon as it is available. *Circulation* • Perform chest compressions. *Defibrillation* • Ensure availability of monitor/defibrillator. ▼
Advanced life support	**Perform Secondary ABCD Survey** • Administer oxygen, establish IV access, attach cardiac monitor, administer fluids as needed (O_2, IV, monitor, fluids).

- Assess vital signs, attach pulse oximeter, and monitor BP.
- Obtain and review 12-lead ECG, portable chest x-ray film.
- Perform a focused history and physical exam.

- Is the patient stable or unstable?
- Is the patient's cardiac function normal or impaired?
- Is the patient experiencing serious signs and symptoms because of the tachycardia?
- Attempt to identify patient's cardiac rhythm using 12-lead ECG, clinical information.
- Is Wolff-Parkinson-White syndrome (WPW) present (e.g., young patient; HR >300; ECG: short PR interval, wide QRS, delta wave)?
- Has WPW been present for > or <48 hours?

Identify the Patient's Cardiac Rhythm

Continued

Wolff-Parkinson-White (WPW) Syndrome Algorithm—cont'd

Normal cardiac function		Impaired cardiac function*	
Onset <48 hr **Control rate**	**Onset >48 hr** **Control rate**	**Onset <48 hr** **Control rate**	**Onset >48 hr** **Control rate**
Cardioversion **or** Amiodarone (IIb) **or** Procainamide (IIb) **or** Flecainide (IIb) **or** Propafenone (IIb) **or** Sotalol (IIb)	Use antiarrhythmics with extreme causation because of embolic risk	Cardioversion **or** Amiodarone (IIb)	Use antiarrhythmics with extreme caution because of embolic risk
Convert rhythm	**Convert rhythm**	**Convert rhythm**	**Convert rhythm**
Cardioversion **or** Amiodarone (IIb) **or** Procainamide (IIb) **or** Flecainide (IIb) **or** Propafenone (IIb) **or** Sotalol (IIb)	Delayed cardioversion **or** Early cardioversion	Cardioversion	Delayed cardioversion **or** Early cardioversion

*Impaired cardiac function = ejection fraction <40% or congestive heart failure.

Delayed cardioversion: Anticoagulation therapy for 3 weeks before cardioversion for at least 48 hours in conjunction with cardioversion and for at least 4 weeks after successful cardioversion.

Early cardioversion: IV heparin immediately, transesophageal echocardiography (TEE) to rule out atrial thrombus, cardioversion within 24 hours anticoagulation × 4 weeks.

Medication Dosing

Amiodarone—150 mg IV bolus over 10 minutes followed by an infusion of 1 mg/min for 6 hours and then a maintenance infusion of 0.5 mg/min. Repeat supplementary infusion of 150 mg as necessary for recurrent or resistant dysrhythmias. Maximum total daily dose 2 g.

Procainamide—100 mg over 5 minutes (20 mg/min). Maximum total dose 17 mg/kg. Maintenance infusion 1-4 mg/min.

Flecainide, propafenone—IV form not currently approved for use in the United States.

Sotalol—1-1.5 mg/kg IV slowly at a rate of 10 mg/min.

Modified from Aehlert B: *ACLS quick review study guide,* ed 2, St Louis, 2001, Mosby, p 441.

Sustained Monomorphic Ventricular Tachycardia

Basic life support	**Perform Primary ABCD Survey** • Correct critical problems *immediately* as they are identified. • Assess responsiveness. • Call for help/Call for defibrillator. *Airway* • Open the airway. *Breathing* • Deliver two slow breaths; administer oxygen as soon as it is available. *Circulation* • Perform chest compressions. *Defibrillation* • Ensure availability of monitor/defibrillator. ▼
Advanced life support	**Perform Secondary ABCD Survey** • Administer oxygen, establish IV access, attach cardiac monitor, administer fluids as needed (O_2, IV, monitor, fluids).

- Assess vital signs, attach pulse oximeter, and monitor BP.
- Obtain and review 12-lead ECG, portable chest x-ray film.
- Perform a focused history and physical exam.

- Is the patient stable or unstable?
- Is the patient experiencing serious signs and symptoms because of the tachycardia?
- Determine if the rhythm is monomorphic or polymorphic VT and determine patient's QT interval.

Identify the Patient's Cardiac Rhythm

Continued

ACLS Guidelines for Adult Emergency Cardiac Care Algorithms

Sustained Monomorphic Ventricular Tachycardia—cont'd

Stable Patient

May proceed directly to synchronized cardioversion, or use one of the following.

Normal cardiac function
- Procainamide (IIa)
- Sotalol (IIa)
- Amiodarone (IIb)
- Lidocaine (IIb)

Impaired cardiac function*
- Amiodarone (IIb)
- Lidocaine (indeterminate)

If medication therapy ineffective, perform synchronized cardioversion.

Unstable VT with a pulse

- If hemodynamically unstable, sync 100 J, 200 J, 300 J, and 360 J, (or equivalent biphasic energy).
- If hypotensive (systolic BP <90), unresponsive, or if severe pulmonary edema exists, defibrillate with same energy.

*Impaired cardiac function = ejection fraction <40% or congestive heart failure.

▼

Medication Dosing

Amiodarone—150 mg IV bolus over 10 minutes. If chemical conversion successful, follow with IV infusion of 1 mg/min for 6 hours and then a maintenance infusion of 0.5 mg/min. Repeat supplementary infusions of 150 mg as necessary for recurrent or resistant dysrhythmias. Maximum total daily dose 2 g.

Lidocaine—1-1.5 mg/kg initial dose. Repeat dose is half the initial dose every 5-10 minutes. Maximum total dose 3 mg/kg. If chemical conversion successful, maintenance infusion 1-4 mg/min. If impaired cardiac function, dose = 0.5-0.75 mg/kg IV push. May repeat every 5-10 minutes. Maximum total dose 3 mg/kg. If chemical conversion successful, maintenance infusion 1-4 mg/min.

Procainamide—100 mg over 5 minutes (20 mg/min). Maximum total dose 17 mg/kg. If chemical conversion successful, maintenance infusion 1-4 mg/min.

Sotalol—1-1.5 mg/kg IV slowly at a rate of 10 mg/min.

Modified from Aehlert B: *ACLS quick review study guide,* ed 2, St Louis, 2001, Mosby, p 443.

Polymorphic Ventricular Tachycardia

Basic life support	**Perform Primary ABCD Survey** • Correct critical problems immediately as they are identified. • Assess responsiveness. • Call for help/Call for defibrillator. *Airway* • Open the airway. *Breathing* • Deliver two slow breaths; administer oxygen as soon as it is available. *Circulation* • Perform chest compressions. *Defibrillation* • Ensure availability of monitor/defibrillator. ▼
Advanced life support	**Perform Secondary ABCD Survey** • Administer oxygen, establish IV access, attach cardiac monitor, administer fluids as needed (O_2, IV, monitor, fluids).

- Assess vital signs, attach pulse oximeter, and monitor BP.
- Obtain and review 12-lead ECG, portable chest x-ray film.
- Perform a focused history and physical exam.

- Is the patient stable or unstable?
- Is the patient experiencing serious signs and symptoms because of the tachycardia?
- Determine if the rhythm is monomorphic or polymorphic VT and determine patient's QT interval.

Identify the Patient's Cardiac Rhythm

Continued

Polymorphic Ventricular Tachycardia—cont'd

Stable Patient

Polymorphic VT Normal QT interval		Polymorphic VT Normal QT Prolonged QT interval (suggests torsades de pointes)	
Normal cardiac function	**Impaired cardiac function***	**Normal cardiac function**	**Impaired cardiac function***
Treat ischemia if present Correct electrolyte abnormalities May proceed directly to electrical therapy or use **one** of the following: Amiodarone (IIb) **or** Lidocaine (IIb) **or** Procainamide (IIb) **or** Sotalol (IIb) **or** Beta-blockers (indeterminate)	May proceed directly to electrical therapy or use **one** of the following: Amiodarone (IIb) **or** Lidocaine (indeterminate)	Discontinue meds that prolong QT Correct electrolyte abnormalities May proceed directly to electrical therapy or use **one** of the following: Magnesium (indeterminate) **or** Overdrive pacing with or without beta-blocker (indeterminate) **or** Isoproterenol (indeterminate) **or** Phenytoin (indeterminate) Lidocaine (indeterminate)	May proceed directly to electrical therapy or use **one** of the following: Amiodarone (IIb) **or** Lidocaine (indeterminate)

*Impaired cardiac function = ejection fraction <40% or congestive heart failure.

If medication therapy ineffective, use electrical therapy.

- Sustained (>30 sec or causing hemodynamic collapse) polymorphic VT should be treated with an unsynchronized shock, using an initial energy of 200 J.
- If unsuccessful, a second shock of 200-300 J should be given and, if necessary, a third shock of 360 J.

Medication Dosing

Amiodarone—150 mg IV bolus over 10 minutes. If chemical conversion successful, follow with IV infusion of 1 mg/min for 6 hours and then a maintenance infusion of 0.5 mg/min. Repeat supplementary infusions of 150 mg as necessary for recurrent or resistant dysrhythmias. Maximum total daily dose 2 g.

Beta-blockers—*Esmolol:* 0.5 mg/kg over 1 minute followed by a maintenance infusion at 50 mcg/kg/min for 4 minutes. If inadequate response, administer a second bolus of 0.5 mg/kg over 1 minute and increase maintenance infusion to 100 mcg/kg/min. The bolus dose (0.5 mg/kg) and titration of the maintenance infusion (addition of 50 mcg/kg/min) can be repeated every 4 minutes to a maximum infusion of 300 mcg/kg/min. *Metoprolol:* 5 mg slow IV push over 5 minutes × 3 as needed to a total dose of 15 mg over 15 minutes. *Atenolol:* 5 mg slow IV (over 5 min). Wait 10 minutes, then give second dose of 5 mg slow IV (over 5 min)

Isoproterenol—Can be used as a temporizing measure until overdrive pacing can be instituted if no evidence of coronary artery disease, ischemic syndromes, or other contraindications; 2-10 mcg/min. Mix 1 mg in 500 mL NS or D5W.

Continued

Polymorphic Ventricular Tachycardia—cont'd

Lidocaine—1-1.5 mg/kg initial dose. Repeat half the initial dose every 5-10 minutes. Maximum total dose 3 mg/kg. If chemical conversion successful, maintenance infusion 1-4 mg/min. If impaired cardiac function, dose = 0.5-0.75 mg/kg IV push. May repeat every 5-10 minutes. Maximum total dose 3 mg/kg. If chemical conversion successful, maintenance infusion 1-4 mg/min.

Magnesium—Loading dose of 1-2 g mixed in 50-100 mL over 5-10 minutes IV. If chemical conversion successful, follow with 0.5-1 g/hr IV infusion.

Phenytoin—250 mg IV at a rate of 25-50 mg/min in NS using a central vein.

Procainamide—100 mg over 5 minutes (20 mg/min). Maximum total dose of 17 mg/kg. If chemical conversion successful, maintenance infusion 1-4 mg/min.

Sotalol—1-1.5 mg/kg IV slowly at a rate of 10 mg/min.

Modified from Aehlert B: *ACLS quick review study guide,* ed 2, St Louis, 2001, Mosby, p 445.

Basic life support	**Perform Primary ABCD Survey**
	• Correct critical problems *immediately* as they are identified.
	• Assess responsiveness.
	• Call for help/Call for defibrillator.
	Airway
	• Open the airway.
	Breathing
	• Deliver two slow breaths; administer oxygen as soon as it is available.
	Circulation
	• Perform chest compressions.
	Defibrillation
	• Ensure availability of monitor/defibrillator.

Continued

Advanced life support	**Perform Secondary ABCD Survey**
	• Administer oxygen, establish IV access, attach cardiac monitor, administer fluids as needed (O_2, IV, monitor, fluids).
	• Assess vital signs, attach pulse oximeter, and monitor BP.
	• Obtain and review 12-lead ECG, portable chest x-ray film.
	• Perform a focused history and physical exam.
	▼
	• Is the patient stable or unstable?
	• Is the patient experiencing serious signs and symptoms because of the tachycardia?
	• Use 12-lead ECG/clinical information to help clarify rhythm diagnosis.
	▼
	Identify the Patient's Cardiac Rhythm

Stable Patient

Rhythm confirmed as SVC	Wide-complex tachycardia of unknown origin		Rhythm confirmed as VT
	Normal cardiac function	Impaired cardiac function*	
Go to narrow-QRS tachycardia algorithm	Sync cardioversion **or** Procainamide (IIb) **or** Amiodarone (IIb)	Sync cardioversion **or** Amiodarone (IIb)	Go to VT algorithm

If medication therapy ineffective, perform synchronized cardioversion.

Unstable Patient

- If hemodynamically unstable, sync 100 J, 200 J, 300 J and 360 J, or equivalent biphasic energy.
- If hypotensive (systolic BP <90), unresponsive, or if severe pulmonary edema exists, defibrillate with same energy.

Continued

Medication Dosing

Amiodarone—150 mg IV bolus over 10 minutes. If chemical conversion successful, follow with IV infusion of 1 mg/min for 6 hours and then a maintenance infusion of 0.5 mg/min. Repeat supplementary infusion of 150 mg as necessary for recurrent or resistant dysrhythmias. Maximum total daily dose 2 g.

Procainamide—100 mg over 5 minutes (20 mg/min). Maximum total dose 17 mg/kg. If chemical conversion successful, maintenance infusion 1-4 mg/min.

Modified from Aehlert B: *ACLS quick review study guide,* ed 2, St Louis, 2001, Mosby, p 449.

Initial Assessment and General Treatment of the Patient With an Acute Coronary Syndrome (ACS)

Initial Assessment
Goal: Targeted clinical exam and 12-lead ECG within 10 minutes.

Prehospital
- Obtain a brief, targeted history/physical exam (determine age, gender; signs/symptoms, pain presentation, including location of pain, duration, quality, relation to effort, time of symptom onset; history of coronary artery disease [CAD]; CAD risk factors present?; and history of Viagra use).
- Assess vital signs, determine oxygen saturation.

If above consistent with possible or definite ACS:
- Use checklist (yes-no); focus on eligibility for reperfusion therapy; evaluate contraindications to aspirin and heparin.
- Establish IV access, ECG monitoring.
- Administer aspirin 162-325 mg (chewed), if no reason for exclusion.
- Obtain 12-lead ECG (machine interpretation or transmission of ECG to physician).
- Draw blood for initial serum cardiac marker levels (to lab on arrival in Emergency Department).

Consider triage to facility capable of angiography and revascularization if any of the following are present:
- Signs of shock
- Pulmonary edema (rales >halfway up)
- Heart rate ≥100 beats/min and SBP ≤100 mm Hg

Continued

Emergency Department
RN TRIAGE FOR RAPID CARE
- Obtain a brief, targeted history/physical exam (determine age, gender; signs/symptoms, pain presentation, including location of pain, duration, quality, relation to effort, time of symptom onset; history of CAD, CAD risk factors present) and history of Viagra use.
- Assess vital signs, determine oxygen saturation.
- Establish IV access, ECG monitoring.
- Obtain 12-lead ECG (present to physician for review).

PHYSICIAN EVALUATION
If above consistent with possible or definite ACS:
- Brief, targeted history/physical exam
- Evaluate eligibility for reperfusion therapy and contraindications to aspirin and heparin.
- Administer aspirin 162-325 mg (chewed); if no reason for exclusion.
- Administer nitroglycerin as indicated.
- Evaluate 12-lead ECG—Categorize patient into one of three groups: ST-elevation or new or presumably new left bundle branch block (LBBB); ST-depression/transient ST-segment/T wave changes; normal or nondiagnostic ECG.
- Obtain serial ECGs in patients with history suggesting myocardial infarction (MI) and nondiagnostic ECG.
- Obtain baseline serum cardiac marker levels (CK-MB, troponin T or I, myoglobin).

- Obtain lab specimens (CBC, lipid profile, electrolytes, coagulation studies).
- Obtain portable chest x-ray film.
- Evaluate results.

GENERAL TREATMENT
- Oxygen 4 L/min by nasal cannula for first 2-3 hours (class IIa).
- Oxygen 4 L/min by cannula, titrate if pulmonary congestion, SaO_2 <90% (class I).
- **Aspirin** 162-325 mg (chewed) (if hypersensitivity exists, ticlopidine); may administer via rectal suppository (325 mg) if nausea, vomiting, upper GI disorder present.
- **Nitroglycerin** sublingual or spray; may repeat twice at 5-min intervals (ensure IV access, SBP >90 mm Hg, HR >50 beats/min, no right ventricular infarction).
- **Morphine** 2-4 mg IV if pain not relieved with nitroglycerin; may repeat every 5 minutes (ensure SBP >90 mm Hg).

Modified from Aehlert B: *ACLS quick review study guide*, ed 2, St Louis, 2001, Mosby, p 450.

Management of ST-Segment Elevation Myocardial Infarction (MI)

ST-segment elevation ≥1 mm in two or more anatomically contiguous leads or new, or presumably new, left bundle branch block (LBBB)
• Confirm diagnosis by signs/symptoms, ECG, serum cardiac markers.

▼

All patients with ST-segment elevation myocardial infarction (MI) should receive the following (if no contraindications):
• **Antiplatelet therapy**—Aspirin 162-325 mg (chewed)
• **Antiischemia therapy**—Beta-blockers, nitroglycerin IV (if ongoing ischemia or uncorrected hypertension)
• **Antithrombin therapy**—Heparin (if using fibrin-specific lytics)
• **ACE inhibitors** (after 6 hr or when stable)—Especially with large or anterior MI, heart failure without hypotension (SBP >1000 mm Hg), previous MI

Symptom onset ≤12 hours			
Patient eligible for reperfusion? (Goals—*Fibrinolytics:* Door-to-drug time <30 min. *Primary PCI:* Door-to-dilation time 90 ± 30 min.)			
Yes		**No**	
Signs of cardiogenic shock or contraindications to fibrinolytics?		Persistent or stuttering symptoms or ECG changes?	
Yes	**No**	**Yes**	**No**
• PCI • Medical management	Can cath lab be mobilized within 60 minutes?	• Cardiac cath • Medical management	• Medical management
	Yes | **No**		
	• PCI | • Fibrinolysis (alteplase, reteplase, strepto-kinase, anistreplase, **or** tenecteplase)		

PCI, Percutaneous coronary intervention (angioplasty ± stent).

Continued

Management of ST-Segment Elevation Myocardial Infarction (MI)—cont'd

Symptom onset >12 hours

Persistent symptoms	Resolution of symptoms
• Consider reperfusion • Medical management	• Medical management

Modified from Aehlert B: *ACLS quick review study guide,* ed 2, St Louis, 2001, Mosby, p 451.

Management of Unstable Angina/Non–ST-Segment Elevation Myocardial Infarction (MI)

ECG changes in two or more anatomically contiguous leads
- ST-segment depression >1 mm or T wave inversion >1 mm **or**
- Transient (<30 min) ST-segment/T wave changes >1 mm with discomfort

Confirm diagnosis by signs/symptoms, ECG, serum cardiac markers.

All patients with unstable angina/non–ST-segment elevation MI should receive the following (if no contraindications)
- **Aspirin**—162-325 mg (chewed) if not already administered (and no contraindications) (antiplatelet therapy).
- **Heparin IV** (antithrombin therapy).

If high-risk patient, give:
- **Aspirin + glycoprotein IIb/IIa inhibitors** (i.e., Integrilin, Aggrastat, ReoPro) + IV heparin **or**
- **Aspirin + glycoprotein IIb/IIa inhibitors + SC low-molecular-weight heparin** (i.e., enoxaparin, [Lovenox], dalteparin [Fragmin])

Continued

Management of Unstable Angina/Non–ST-Segment Elevation Myocardial Infarction (MI)—cont'd

High-risk criteria
- Persistent ("stuttering") symptoms/recurrent ischemia; left ventricular (LV) dysfunction, congestive heart failure (CHF); widespread ECG changes; prior MI, positive troponin or CK-MB.

Antiischemic therapy (e.g., metoprolol, atenolol, esmolol, propranolol) includes:
- **Beta-blockers**—If patient not previously on beta-blockers or inadequately treated on current dose of beta-blocker (if no contraindications).
- **Nitroglycerin** sublingual tablet or spray, followed by IV nitroglycerin—if symptoms persist despite sublingual nitroglycerin therapy and initiation of beta-blocker therapy (and SBP >90 mm Hg).
- **Morphine**—2-4 mg IV (if discomfort is not relieved or symptoms recur despite antiischemic therapy); may repeat every 5 minutes (ensure SBP >90 Hg).

Assess clinical status: Is patient clinically stable?	
Yes	**No**
Continue in-hospital observation Consider stress testing	Cardiac cath • If anatomy suitable for revascularization: PCI, CABG • If anatomy unsuitable: Medical management

PCI, Percutaneous coronary intervention; *CABG,* coronary artery bypass grafting.
Modified from Aehlert B: *ACLS quick review study guide,* ed 2, St Louis, 2001, Mosby, p 452.

Management of Patient With a Suspected Acute Coronary Syndrome and Nondiagnostic or Normal ECG

- Evaluate signs/symptoms, serial ECGs, serum cardiac markers.
- Administer aspirin + other therapy as appropriate.
- Assess patient's clinical risk or death/nonfatal MI.
- Perform a focused history and physical exam.
- Obtain follow-up serum cardiac marker levels, serial ECG monitoring.
- Consider evaluation and treatment in Emergency Department, chest pain unit, or monitored bed.
- Consider radionuclide, echocardiography.

Modified from Aehlert B: *ACLS quick review study guide,* ed 2, St Louis, 2001, Mosby, p 453.

Management of Acute Pulmonary Edema

Basic life support	**Perform Primary ABCD Survey** • Correct critical problems *immediately* as they are identified. • Assess responsiveness. • Call for help/Call for defibrillator. *Airway* • Open the airway. *Breathing* • Deliver two slow breaths; administer oxygen as soon as it is available. *Circulation* • Perform chest compressions. *Defibrillation* • Ensure availability of monitor/defibrillator. ▼

| Advanced life support | **Perform Secondary ABCD Survey**
• Obtain arterial blood gas before oxygen administration if possible.
• Administer oxygen, establish IV access, attach cardiac monitor, administer fluids as needed (O_2, IV, monitor).
• Assess vital signs, attach pulse oximeter, and monitor BP.
• Obtain and review 12-lead ECG, portable chest x-ray film.
• Perform a focused history and physical exam. |

Continued

If feasible and BP permits, place patient in sitting position with feet dependent:
- Increases lung volume and vital capacity
- Decreases work of respiration
- Decreases venous return, decreases preload

If systolic BP >100 mm Hg:
- **Sublingual nitroglycerin**—1 tablet or spray every 5 minutes (max 3 tablets) until IV nitroglycerin or nitroprusside can take effect.
- **Furosemide IV**—0.5-1.0 mg/kg (typically 20-40 mg) (can repeat in 30 min if symptoms persist and BP stable).
- Consider **morphine IV**—2-4 mg.

Consider additional preload/afterload reduction—nitroglycerin or nitroprusside IV, angiotensin converting enzyme (ACE) inhibitors (if SBP >100 mm Hg):
- **Nitroglycerin IV**—Start at 5 mcg/min and increase gradually until mean systolic pressure falls by 10%-15%, avoid hypotension (SBP <90 mm Hg) **or**
- **Nitroprusside IV**—0.1-5 mcg/kg/min

Evaluate early for:

- Readily reversible cause: Institute appropriate intervention (e.g., cardiac dysrhythmias, tamponade).
- Myocardial ischemia/infarction: Institute appropriate intervention-candidate for fibrinolytic therapy? PTCA?

If patient is refractory to previous therapies, hypotensive, or in cardiogenic shock:

- Consider fluid or **IV inotropic** and/or **vasopressor** agents (e.g., dobutamine, dopamine, norepinephrine).
- Consider pulmonary and systemic arterial catheterization.
- Obtain ECG to assist in diagnosis, evaluation, and reparability of culprit lesion or condition.
- Consider need for mechanical circulatory assistance (balloon pump).

Modified from Aehlert B: *ACLS quick review study guide,* ed 2, St Louis, 2001, Mosby, p 454.

Management of Hypotension/Shock: Suspected Pump Problem

Basic life support	**Perform Primary ABCD Survey** • Correct critical problems *immediately* as they are identified. • Assess responsiveness. • Call for help/Call for defibrillator. *Airway* • Open the airway. *Breathing* • Deliver two slow breaths; administer oxygen as soon as it is available. *Circulation* • Perform chest compressions. *Defibrillation* • Ensure availability of monitor/defibrillator. ▼

| Advanced life support | **Perform Secondary ABCD Survey**
- Administer oxygen, establish IV access, attach cardiac monitor, administer fluids as needed (O_2, IV, monitor, fluids).
- Assess vital signs, attach pulse oximeter, and monitor BP.
- Obtain and review 12-lead ECG, portable chest x-ray film.
- Perform a focused history and physical exam.

Continued |

Hypotension—Suspected Pump Problem
- If breath sounds are clear, consider fluid challenge of 250-500 mL NS to ensure adequate ventricular filling pressure before **vasopressor** administration.

Marked Hypotension (Systolic BP <70 mm Hg)/Cardiogenic Shock
Pharmacologic management:
- **Norepinephrine infusion**—0.5-30 mcg/min until SBP 80 mm Hg.
- Then attempt to change to **dopamine**—5-15 mcg/kg/min until SBP 90 mm Hg.
- **Dobutamine IV**—2-20 mcg/kg/min can be given simultaneously in an attempt to reduce magnitude of dopamine infusion.
Consider balloon pump or patient transfer to a cardiac interventional facility.

Moderate Hypotension (Systolic BP 70-90 mm Hg)
- **Dopamine**—5-15 mcg/kg/min.
- If BP remains low despite dopamine doses >20 mcg/kg/min, may substitute **norepinephrine** in doses of 0.5-30 mcg/min.
- Once SBP ≥90 with dopamine, add **dobutamine** 2-20 mcg/kg/min and attempt to taper off dopamine.

Systolic BP ≥90 mm Hg
- **Dobutamine**—2-20 mcg/kg/min.

▼

Medication Dosing
Norepinephrine IV—0.5-30 mcg/min
Dopamine IV—5-15 mcg/kg/min
Dobutamine IV—2-20 mcg/kg/min

Modified from Aehlert B: *ACLS quick review study guide,* ed 2, St Louis, 2001, Mosby, p 455.

Management of Hypotension/Shock: Suspected Volume Problem

| Basic life support | **Perform Primary ABCD Survey**
• Correct critical problems *immediately* as they are identified.
• Assess responsiveness.
• Call for help/Call for defibrillator.

Airway
• Open the airway.

Breathing
• Deliver two slow breaths; administer oxygen as soon as it is available.

Circulation
• Perform chest compressions.

Defibrillation
• Ensure availability of monitor/defibrillator.

▼ |

Advanced life support	**Perform Secondary ABCD Survey** • Administer oxygen, establish IV access, attach cardiac monitor, administer fluids as needed (O_2, IV, monitor, fluids). • Assess vital signs, attach pulse oximeter, and monitor BP. • Obtain and review 12-lead ECG, portable chest x-ray film. • Perform a focused history and physical exam. **Hypotension: Suspected Volume (or Vascular Resistance) Problem** • Volume replacement. • Fluid challenge (250-500 mL IV boluses—reassess). • Blood transfusion (if appropriate). • If cause known, institute appropriate intervention (e.g., septic shock, anaphylaxis). • Consider **vasopressors,** if indicated, to improve vascular tone if no response to fluid challenge(s).

Modified from Aehlert B: *ACLS quick review study guide,* ed 2, St Louis, 2001, Mosby, p 456.

Basic life support	**Perform Primary ABCD Survey**
	• Correct critical problems *immediately* as they are identified.
	• Assess responsiveness.
	• Call for help/Call for defibrillator.
	Airway
	• Open the airway.
	Breathing
	• Deliver two slow breaths; administer oxygen as soon as it is available.
	Circulation
	• Perform chest compressions.
	Defibrillation
	• Ensure availability of monitor/defibrillator.
	▼

| Advanced life support | **Perform Secondary ABCD Survey**
- Administer oxygen, establish IV access, attach cardiac monitor, administer fluids as needed (O_2, IV, monitor, fluids).
- Assess vital signs, attach pulse oximeter, and monitor BP.
- Obtain and review 12-lead ECG, portable chest x-ray film.
- Perform a focused history and physical exam.

Hypotension: Suspected Rate Problem
- *If rate too slow:* Bradycardia algorithm.
- *If rate too fast:* Determine width of QRS, then use appropriate tachycardia algorithm. |

Modified from Aehlert B: *ACLS quick review study guide,* ed 2, St Louis, 2001, Mosby, p 456.

Index

Index

Index

Index

Index

Index